Exposing the Demon

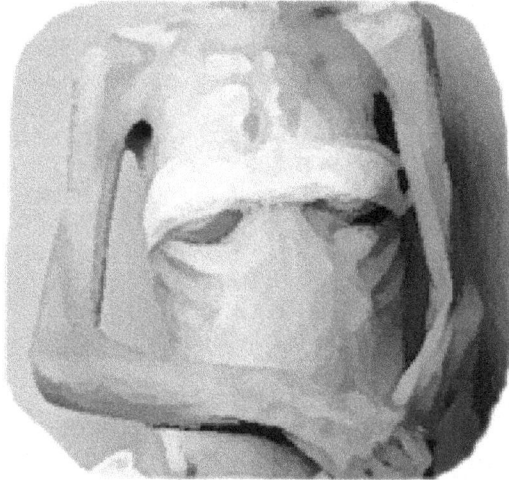

the true nature of an *eating disorder*
and what you can do to defeat it

by Alissa Hall

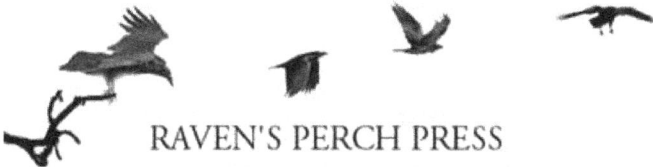

RAVEN'S PERCH PRESS
"Thoughts are things and words have wings."

EXPOSING THE DEMON:

the true nature of an eating disorder
and what you can do to defeat it

by Alissa Hall

Library of Congress Cataloging-in-Publication Data
Hall, Alissa.
Exposing the Demon: the true nature of an eating disorder and what you can do to defeat it /
by Alissa Hall.
1. Anorexia nervosa.
2. Eating disorders.

ISBN: 978-0-6151-6203-4
Printed in the U.S.A.

Author's Note: The intentional use of capitals within the narrative is meant to express archetypal concepts that reach beyond the circumstance of a sufferer's life to a more universal understanding for all readers.

Quotation from The Chicken Qabalah of Rabbi Lamed Ben Clifford is used expressly with Lon Milo DuQuette's permission.

Cover design by Alissa Hall

For more writings and illustrations by Alissa Hall, please visit:
WWW.ALISSAHALL.COM

"Darkness cannot drive out darkness; only light can do that. Hate cannot drive out hate; only love can do that."

– Dr. Martin Luther King, Jr.

"What is that within us which does sound a trumpet and all that is lower in our nature rises in response—almost in a moment, almost in the twinkling of an eye."

- Arthur E. Waite, on the Judgement card, <u>The Pictorial Key to the Tarot</u>

෨Welcome to Hell ෬

Let us begin right here, right where the Demon does not wish us to. Take this... it's a very powerful Flashlight for you to keep, and you're gonna need it. I know, the instructions are foreign–you can't even figure out how to turn the Flashlight on yet. Don't worry about that. I'm here, and I do know how. And, I can try to teach you. From this point forward, you and I will tell ourselves that every step along this road belongs to no one but you... and me. There are no rules but those we decide to make together. After all, there have been enough Rules.

Here's the deal... this place? This claustrophobic mental space of confinement and pain you've been living in for so long? This isn't new to me. I've been down this road too–it's an ugly one, isn't it? So barren and dry, so bereft of... hope. Of Love. The Demon is very comfortable in this place; this is *exactly* how the Demon likes it.

So, guess what the Demon hates? The Demon hates the fact that I'm about to turn on this bigass Flashlight of mine, and show you the Truth of how ugly It really is. After that, it will be your turn–your Flashlight will expose your Demon, and you'll need a weapon to keep It at bay. That weapon is the Light of Truth. All Demons hate the Light.

Let's be clear from the beginning, I can't fight your fight. No one else can. But, that doesn't mean I can't help you. Although, I bet your Demon told you that "no one can help you" once or twice along the way, didn't It?

Perhaps you're reading these words and you are not in the Demon's grip, but your wife, your sister, your daughter is... and she's dying before your eyes. You've tried everything and still don't know what to do. The Demon has learned to make you helpless, as helpless and fearful as it has made the one whom It controls. I *know* you want to help the one you love who is suffering so intensely. This book may talk directly to the sufferer, but in doing so, let it teach you how to talk to the one you love.

Let me tell you the worst part. The Demon doesn't want to let go; not of me, and not of you... not ever. The Demon is the rat who is happy to go down with the sinking ship. The Demon is the master manipulator, and the second I begin to shine my Flashlight on yours, It'll hit every panic button It can as It tries to skitter back into the darkness, like a cockroach seeking the comfort of shadows. As soon as you see It for the repulsive thing It is... next, It will turn that message of disgust against you and me... because we're the ones holding the Flashlights.

So, be ready. Be ware. But, do not give the Demon the banquet of your fear; It's not nearly as big or as badass as you think. It just tells you so. Another lie.

I am not a doctor. I am not a nutritionist. I am not a psychiatrist or psychologist. I am, by all Westernized standards, unqualified to offer you this manual of help. Your own Demon may soon remind you of all these things as It points Its finger to me and lies about how I'm a hack, and I don't know what I'm talking about.

I *know* how the Demon will react; I *know* how to talk Its talk. The Demon was my best friend for years, and we got very comfortable with each other back in the day. But now? Now it means I can often guess Its messages so accurately people flinch.

"How did you know I've been saying that in my head? How did you know I was just thinking that?" I listened to the Demon for years and I know It so well, that's how. The Demon spoke to me all day, every day. How could I *not* know?

That knowing keeps me a half-step ahead of It more often than It likes, now that I'm no longer on Its side. So, let's start right here, lost in the midst of your own personal hell. I'm the tour guide down here, my dearest, and I'm here to help you try to find your way back.

See, I know damn well what I'm talking about, and, unlike so many others of us who are also facing the Demon, I'm a writer. I have the words to tell others, and you know what, Demon? I'm already breaking the first golden Rule you ever made me obey, I'm Telling On You. I'm going to use bad grammar and poor English, and maybe even a few cuss words along the way if I have to, because that's what we do in real life when we talk to each other.

I wrote this book to try to talk to *you*, my unknown sister, in hope of helping. Herein, I will often address you as a she, but let us *never* believe this is a phenomenon that only females encounter. The Demon hides in our brothers' minds also, and with them It festers under the Gender Lie, keeping these men silent with the shame and humiliation It continues to inflict by insisting this is a Girl's Problem. That a Real Man wouldn't behave or act this way.

I know, I know. The list of lies the Demon can come up with is yeah-long, but essentially… It's always saying the exact same thing.

I was once exactly as you are. I am *still* as you are. But, in many important ways, I am not. I learned a lot along the way.

In this work, you're *not* going to hear about psychological issues with your mother, or the inability to accept your womanhood, or trying to hold on to your girlhood by stopping your body from menstruating–those tired theories have plagued us, the true sufferers, for decades. You *are* going to hear me talk about some metaphysical ideas on emotions and personal energy, the Authentic Self, and thought forms, and you might wonder what the hell I'm getting at, and why should anyone believe this kooky, airyfairy bullcrap when there's no proof of the stuff she's dishing anyhow?

More Demon talk. The Demon wants to shut down any conversation, and therefore any analysis, of It every moment It can. And so, It says whatever It must to try and get the conversation to simply STOP!

But, I'm not stopping. I'm not afraid of the Demon any more. I *will* tell you. It's what I learned, and it's helped others like us simply to hear it. Others who have asked me, "You said you got over your eating disorder, Alissa. How did you do it?"

They ask me the same question I had asked of other recovered ones while still in the depths of my own personal suffering. And now, when they ask *me,* in their eyes I see the last glimmer of hope not yet extinguished, not yet drowned by the Demon's hate.

I say to you now what was once said to me in the midst of my own despair, "There is a path back."

And, buried deeply inside, I yet remember how it felt, while still suffering, to wonder… how? How? Please, you've gotta tell me now, cuz I don't think I can last much longer in here…. How did you do this?

Right here, right now–I'll tell you how. I've told others the keys I used to confront my Demon, and I can tell you all I learned to try and help you. My best friend Autumn has a saying, if the suffering I've endured helps one person later in life then at least somehow it was worth it.

My eating disorder required first that I learn the lessons I needed about myself and now, as I continue to defeat It, I help others when they've asked me for help. That's because I know how to speak up, to be the Voice for the one who cannot yet speak. This is how I continue to fight my Demon. I use my words, I use my Voice. I break Rule Number One and flaunt the fact in my Demon's face, laughing at It the way It once laughed and mocked me.

I'm not here to guarantee your success. I *will* show you the tools that no one else could give to me, the ones I found and put together on my own. I had to find them by reading books, talking with friends, through my meditations and prayers, conversations with my guardian angels (my Teachers, or spirit guides), and my larger relationship to Divinity. At no point will I ask you to convert the faith of your heart–myself, I am a Hindu and do not believe in the practice of "religious conversion." So keep your faith, whatever it is, as long as it is your Truth, and I will tell you mine, nothing more.

The cover of this book will tell you it is about "eating disorders." First off, that's a big crock of shit. The disorder you and I have suffered from? It has nothing to do with eating, and we both know it, don't we? The food, the fat grams, the scale, the baggy clothes, the thinspo, the number of bones you can count in your ribcage on any given day… metaphors. Very deeply engrained metaphors. You can deny it for now, if you wish. I don't mind.

My friend Dan later chided me. "You don't *have* an eating disorder!" he insisted. "You have a *thinking* disorder."

I'll say it again. Anorexia, bulimia, overeating? These problems aren't *about* eating, and they never were. They also aren't caused by fashion magazines. They aren't about supermodels, and the "societal pressure to maintain a certain body image in order to be socially acceptable."

The people who make these hypotheses, those who say these things? They are the non-sufferers. They have no idea, my dear. When looking at this disease, they are in the same darkness we are… but their Flashlights are not nearly as high in wattage as the ones that you and I have each got in our beautiful and capable hands, right now.

You may need to take your time while reading this. You may need to take breaks, put the book down while your eyes continue to adjust to the Light. If you're taken with the idea, I recommend starting a journal where you can record along the way anything relevant to your own journey back. It can help tremendously to have one very safe and non-judgmental place to finally begin the process of expunging the toxic messages that right now you can barely admit to hearing inside, not even to yourself.

You may feel Fear along the way. Know this now… the Fear is the Demon's because It knows when It's been caught. The Real You is okay, but you may begin to feel quite shaky at times when old paradigms and thought processes begin to crumble. That's extremely normal, and ultimately very good. So do not let it paralyze you.

I'm going to tell you a lot of things that you may initially reject. Believe it or not, I also initially rejected the realizations as they first came to me. My Demon tried to deny them, and deny them, and deny them. After a while though they just continued to make sense, no matter how long I tried. Still, it's your choice, and it's up to you. Reject away, if that is your wish. I know how easy and preferable it is to keep up the fight, of choosing instead to maintain the daily False Front of the Strong and the Dutiful and the Good.

Wait, that hurt a little to hear, didn't it?

That's because I just said something the Demon once taught me I couldn't say, and I'll bet It's taught the same to you as well. I said this disorder is about "pretending" to be Good, instead of authentically believing in it. I just admitted that even though you bow to Its every demand, the Demon still isn't keeping Its word, still isn't making you feel better. Only much *much* worse. Weaker, and smaller, and uglier, more and more pathetic, until at last, there is almost nothing of the Real You left at all for anyone to find, ever, although my God, I'm dying! Why can't anyone help me in here?

I know the pain—the Demon was my best friend for many years. I lived in this same hell from ages 15 to 28; for years, I did what you did. I believed the lie. I hated my body, I yearned for control. I wanted to be Perfect. A few more pounds lost would fix everything—then I'd feel better about myself. I'd stop the Voice Inside that beat the crap outta me every day.

I believed the Demon's lies... and followed Its rules until the day I realized I would either kill myself from the internal pain, or I could try to finally break free. No one else got me to that point; I got fed up all by myself. And that's individual. Until the victim is *truly* fed up with living with the Demon, no amount of talking or sympathy will make a difference. This I know too. But... you are reading this. You are reaching out, if only a little... if in the only way your Demon will let you.

If you are like me, you picked up this book for the same reason I had for reading multitudinous volumes of books on eating disorders for so many years myself—reading and reading what others had to say in the hope of finding out what was so *wrong* with me, and why I was so incredibly *horrible,* both to myself and to others?

You are lost right now. You feel that a part of you is constantly trying and never succeeding—every day, another set of Hoops to leap through: check the scale, exercise harder, work out longer, eat less, eat less than less, check the scale again. Check the scale after you pee, before you shower, after you shower, if your hair is wet or dry, if your clothes are on or off, if it's morning-weight, just-ate weight, before-bed or middle-of-the-night weight and how does it compare to the weight of last week, of yesterday, of an hour ago, of a few minutes ago? Then, go check the scale again.

Your Demon likes Hoops, mine does too. Your Demon knows, like mine, that as long as It keeps you and I jumping through these stupid little Hoops, we're too busy and too exhausted to really think about anything else, anything important–anything like... It.

As you read, some examples or behaviors I describe may *not* fit your own situation but may speak to another's. No one can duplicate your experiences, but each of us can relate to the shared experience of hosting the Demon inside. It takes on many forms, as individualistic as we are, since we are the ones who created It.

As a result, I do not have a neat formula to give you to make you "better" because there isn't one. I only intend to tell you some realizations I had along this path as I first crawled, then dragged, limped and stumbled my way to something Healthy, something normal, once again. I *didn't* dance my way back. Good health didn't come all at once, but when each realization struck that would assist me to getting closer to being healthy… like Paul at Damascus, the lightning bolt of Truth was impossible to later deny.

Your Demon has taught you to hate yourself, and you've become very good at that task, haven't you?

Don't pretend to be shocked. I know… it's okay. I did the same.

I was the *best* at hating myself. It was the only thing my Demon let me feel pride in. At my lowest, in my mid-twenties, I really excelled at the art. No one on this Earth was as Bad, or as big of a Failure, as me. I had just finished my Bachelor's degree in English, graduating *cum laude*. I had a beautiful new marriage to a man whom I'd loved for years, a home we had bought together and plans to start a family someday. I was a semi-professional ballet and modern dancer who prided herself in her growing art. I worked a full time job with the local library, and was considered beyond capable to the point of sheer diligence at every task given to me.

And yet….

Nothing I ever *ever* did was going to erase the monumental pile of crap that made up my life. But I could try to even out the scales; I could *try*, promised the Demon. "Here's how you can begin to make up for all the problems and trouble you are, you disgusting little pig," said my Demon in Its most loving voice.

And, the Demon handed me an identity, a behavior, a "way out" It promised. It showed me the logic of punishing myself, my mind and my body, as a way to just *begin* to try and make up for all the bad things I intrinsically was.

No good deed of mine would ever be good enough. No A+ was ever plussed enough; nothing I accomplished would ever *ever* live up to what my Demon expected of me.

Does this mean someone with a Demon who dropped out of school, had a child out of wedlock and became addicted to drugs deserves their eating disorder more than I do? Of course not. This book isn't about judgment. Each of us has walked a path of pain and mental anguish that our Demon inflicted upon us. In this, we can realize our mutual strength and support.

How many times have you said to yourself, "You're worthless. You can't do anything right; you have screwed up everything in your entire life, and you have no one but yourself to blame for it. You'll never have any friends, you fucking fatty, and you're never going to succeed. You're built to fail, and I'm going to sit here and laugh while continually watching you do so?"

I know, the Demon goes on and on. I stopped there, because you see? The messages of the Demon? The messages don't change. They can't, the Demon isn't powerful enough to do that... but I am getting beyond myself by discussing the nature of this thing. There will be time for that.

For now, here is your Flashlight.

Go ahead. Switch it on. Don't be afraid, I'm right here with you. See? Here's my hand.

You are not Alone.

ಝNaming the Demonಢ

Last night, there was a news report on ABC about the sky-rocketing number of middle-aged women being diagnosed with eating disorders. And the news caster put on her most compassionate face while telling the viewers of "the pressure more and more middle-aged women are feeling to look thin."

I had to shake my head. It actually *hurts* me to hear the false theories on eating disorders get repeated like rhetoric over and over, as if they were the gospel truth. Ask any sufferer, she'll tell you if she can—it isn't *really* about trying to look like someone else for social acceptance. It isn't even about being Thin.

And yet, if you ask one of us who's hurting, "Then what is it?" we will shrug, stymied. The darkness in here is very thick, and if you have no Flashlight, no beacon of Truth, you simply can't answer because you can't figure it out either.

I will not use the term "eating disorder" often; instead, I will call it by the name I have given it, the Demon. And, there are many reasons why I call it so.

If you could crack open the head of someone under the spell of the Demon she would tell you, if she could, "All day long, all I hear in my head is how horrible I am. How ugly, and fat, and pathetic, and worthless. It's like a nonstop tape that plays and plays—it never lets up, and the moment I begin to feel free of it, it comes smashing back into me. I can't figure out what to do, and I don't know why I'm hurting myself like this, except you have to believe me when I say… it's all I know how to do in order to stay strong."

"Stay strong?" asks the non-Demoned. "You're *starving!* You're so thin you can barely turn a corner without getting light-headed and your electrolytes have plummeted into nonexistence due to all the purging! You're already so weak you could *die!* Don't you get it?"

Let us stop… right here. Get your Flashlight, it's time. You can squeeze my hand as hard as you need to if you get scared. You won't hurt me, I promise. It's the Demon's fear you're feeling right now; It knows when It's being outted.

Most often, when the non-afflicted tries to reason with someone under the Demon's influence, they begin to argue. They get angry; they may get in our faces in the hope that Tough Love will shake us out of it. But, what they can never know is we are already dealing with the most vicious of arguments, all day long, playing inside our heads much louder and more effectively than any raised voice of theirs can ever hope to match. The Demon's voice.

Once, while in the midst of my Demon's grip, my boss said to me, with a concerned frown, "You're starting to look too thin, Alissa." In hindsight, I know what she was trying to say, what she was trying to do. She was trying to help, to start a dialogue, to *do something*. It's awful for the non-afflicted to sit by and watch as we begin the process of mental flagellation, and continue on with the self-abuse by starvation, by binging. It's awkward to begin a conversation with someone who is in complete denial.

But, you know what I heard? Know how my Demon translated this message of concern and Love? "You're *starting* to look thin! You've just barely *begun!* You fat pig, you've barely scratched the surface. You have *so* much further to go, you lazy piece of shit."

And, right behind that thought of self-hatred was the nasty, emotional striking-out against the Love she tried to show me. I thought (but did not say) to my boss, "You haven't even *seen* thin yet, bitch."

That's how my Demon talked. I'd bet real money yours says much the same. How do I know? Like I said, Demons never change.

So repeat it again, Alissa... *you cannot argue or bully a person out of an eating disorder.* You cannot help to reason or logic their way out of it either. Any fight you begin to show, any resistance, and the Demon inside will begin to fight too. Like a person who is possessed, It will use the mouths and words of the one who is suffering to do Its battle.

If confronted, It may use the rest of the body and become physically violent in Its attempts at defense. Often, loved ones have said, "I can't believe the nasty things she's said about me! How can she possibly feel this way about us/our family/our home when we've always given her so much? She actually *hit* me!"

Never, NEVER make the mistake of thinking you're talking to the one you love if they are in the midst of an eating disorder. You *are* talking to their Demon. Their Demon controls their mouths and words, as much as It controls their actions, and It tells them what they are *allowed* to say, and NOT allowed to say.

And the silencing always comes first.

Let's start with the primary Rule every Demon gives us, Rule Number One: You Cannot Say Anything, No One Must Know. You *cannot* ask for help. You are Alone in this. No one can know how much you're hurting, *not ever*. The afflicted cannot ask for help because they are Forbidden to let anyone in that close. Why? The afflicted may not realize it, but the Demon does. It knows that if another person comes close, if another is let inside your heart and mind, It may begin to lose Its psychological hold on the host.

Even if part of the Real Person inside can rationally realize they are dying, or at least heading down a road to terrible self-destruction, they often simply will not say anything, or will vehemently deny the existence of any problems, if asked. They are obeying their Demon's Rules.

And, they're Forbidden from even *telling* you of the *existence* of these Rules that they are living by. The Demon knows no one else can argue or dispute the Rules if the Rules aren't discussed, which means no one can usurp Its power over controlling the host.

The Demon likes the comfort of the dark, of silence. "Hello darkness, my old friend. I've come to talk with you again." It hides Its true nature in secrets, and seeks to keep the Authentic Self just as hidden, while conducting the body and mind on one long and terrible downhill slide.

Getting angry at someone with an eating disorder, getting in their faces will evoke one of two responses… they will either lash out with the force of the Demon in defense, or they will clam up, and go back to Rule Number One: You Cannot Say Anything, and under no circumstances are you allowed to become weak, or to admit you're hurting terribly. You must act Tough and Strong. Use Anger and Silence as your sword and shield if you must.

The image here is the Authentic Self with her hands tied, and a gag over her lips, having been locked inside a dark cage. If she knew how to remove the gag, she would already be screaming for help.

The Demon knows this. It silences us first, because It knows that silence and solitude provide the optimum environment to create the kind of Pain that It needs to continue to grow.

The Rules don't stop there... because you cannot admit how much pain is hidden behind that glowing smile and too-bright eyes, the practice of putting up False Fronts becomes normalcy; we pretend our way through our lives. False Fronts feel intimately necessary on a primal emotional level, because by now the Demon has grown enough in form to manipulate your emotions and continue Its energetic feast. The idea of *not* keeping up your Front is too frightening to consider, so we pretend everything is just fine, that we are Good Girls, and we hide the compulsive behaviors and self-hate, which subtly reinforces the messages of shame and humiliation the Demon has already introduced.

The Demon has convinced you that if any one knew the Real You and how awful you were, they would be horrified. They would most certainly leave, if not right away, they would over time... and then there would be no one but the Demon left in your life. And, nothing could be worse than that.

It creates a state of inherent Fear, and then seeks to *keep* you in it.

It also knows that the Compassion and Love that could be shown to you if you admitted you were hurt and scared, that quality of loving emotions would begin to poison the Demon quickly. And, It can't have that. So, It insists You Cannot Be Weak.

Rule Number Three: The only way to feel good about yourself is to be Perfect. The Demon demands Perpetual Perfection with the hidden promise that once we've achieved this mystical state, we will feel the happiness that is lacking inside right now. This leads us back to the tangle of False Fronts, because we know how imperfect we truly are, the Demon never lets us forget *that*.

Eating disorder sufferers are often highly intelligent, some of the brightest, most capable minds among us all—and yet, when others are judging us, we don't care about the A+'s they give to us. No amount of praise can erase the Demon's messages playing in our head. That's why we try harder, and harder. Many of us are over-achievers by our nature, and the Demon exploits that characteristic to Its own insidious advantage.

The Demon "helps" us achieve the Rule of Perpetual Perfection by showing us the way to reach that unattainably high and oh-so-temptingly close pinnacle—It introduces a behavior. Overeating, starving, purging… those are the most common behaviors for us.

But, and this is important… not *every* self-destructive behavior from a Demon addresses the attempt to achieve Perfection. The self-destructive behavior itself can manifest in various forms, that is, *as any addiction (drugs, alcohol, sex) or any mental compulsion (eating disorders, depression, inherent rage) that begins to "run the vehicle" of the human host.*

Each self-destructive behavior begins the same way each time… with the false promise of This Behavior Will Make Everything that Hurts Inside Go Away. And then, the Demon hands the behavior to us. The behavior can be alcoholism, it can be heroin addiction; it can be an eating disorder.

Here, too often, we see the Hoops begin to form that we must repeat to keep the Demon's daily demands at bay—the ongoing cycles of eating and purging, or non-eating, or overeating, as well as compulsive exercising, and obsession with calories and the scale. A junkie has his daily fix to attend to, that's his Hoop. And, we have ours.

We make bargains with It all day long, because the Demon likes to entertain Itself this way in order to create more Pain. "If I do 100 more sit ups, then I'll have burned enough calories that I can stop and study for a while." Not good enough is the Demon's typical answer, one that only we can hear. *You ate bread with butter on it, do 100 more crunches, and then maybe we'll call it even.*

The Hoops. The Rules. I've never met a Demon who didn't adore Rules. Rules give the Demon more power, an infrastructure. The fact that the Demon's Rules don't make much sense if you really examined them doesn't matter. After all, we don't talk about them, right? We quietly and secretly adopt them in the desperate hope that if we are Good and simply Obey, the Demon will keep Its word and the Pain will begin to subside.

What other kinds of Rules are there, the non-afflicted may ask? Millions. Rules about what foods you can eat, Rules about what foods you can't, Rules about *when* you can eat and when you can't, Rules about how soon you have to throw up afterwards, Rules about calorie consumption, Rules about how long you have to exercise, and the Rules... they just keep changing. But, never to our benefit. The Rules change when the Demon ups the ante, sets the mark up another notch, knowing our over-achiever nature is sure to rise to the bait of the Demon's challenge—*now you have to do twice as much today, and eat half the amount!*

Demons love Pain and Fear, they love despondency. They literally exist on it. It seems paradoxical, but the Demon *knows* Its hurting you, and yet promises to be the one to end your Pain, but not until you've completed the task at hand. Not until you're Worthy.

You'll stop hurting once you're another few pounds thinner. Then, you'll be a good enough person, so good that I'll stop calling you so many names every day. You'll feel so much better about everything *if you could just lose 10 more pounds. In the next two weeks. Or in less time that that. Less would be better.*

Tears and starvation, and ten pounds later we find the Demon has broken Its word... yet again. This is the Cycle of Self-Destruction. It's never-ending, and right here is where so many of us get stuck because we've always believed what the Demon's said. And we believed it because we thought it was coming from ourselves... that is, because we thought there was no difference between "the Demon" and "the Real Me."

But the Demon is the Great Liar.

Over and over, the non-Demoned ask, *why* are you starving yourself? The terrible truth is, because my Demon promised me it would make me feel better, but I'm just not quite there. I've got to work harder, you see... if I just lost a few *more* pounds....

The starvation, the binging… these are coping mechanisms that the Demon introduces into the host's behaviors. They aren't from us, they weren't part of us and they never were. I'll bet you can't really answer *why* you first threw up. Or, *why* you first decided to go an entire day with only four bites consumed. You just started doing it, right? That's because those behaviors *didn't* come from the Real You, they came from the Demon.

Ah, you remember that now. I see the Light beginning to dance in your eyes, my precious one.

Right about now, the non-Demoned are scratching their heads and saying, "really?" Yes, really. Send her to shrinks, ask her a thousand times and she'll still say each time, "I don't *know* why I started doing this, I just kinda thought about it, and then I did it!"

The behaviors are given an ideal place to fester as silence and obedience to the Demon continue to be the only acceptable options we know. Any hope of finding another way to deal with this Pain is quickly put down by the Demon; any glimmer of Hope is rapidly extinguished, all by using variations on the Demon's same metamessage: *You aren't worth helping. You're not* sick *enough, or* thin *enough yet to deserve any help. Why should anyone bother to help you when you're only gonna go right back to throwing up anyhow? You're hopeless!*

So, if you can't talk about it, can't admit you're hurting, and can't ask for help, what do you do? Do you do it alone? And, what the hell DO you do, what is the first step to exorcising this Demon?

Ask a priest, or just rent a scary movie and you'll know the answer… what's the first step in any exorcism? You Call the Demon Out. You give it a name, and thereby you begin to control that which has controlled the host.

You dissociate the host from the parasite.

Here… let me dim my Flashlight a little, I see you squinting. Too much Light all at once is painful. Let us baby-step our way back into it instead.

"What in the hell does that mean, Alissa? Call the Demon out and give it a name?"

It means... listen, my love...

It means... you are *not* the Demon.

You are *not* the one in your head who is saying these things, calling you those names, making those accusations, and telling those lies. You are *not* the one who is bending her knee and habitually sticking her fingernail into the back of her throat in a vain attempt to win an unwinnable war. We'll examine what It *really* is more later, but for now... believe me when I say, the Demon ISN'T the Authentic Self—It doesn't talk like the Authentic Self, It doesn't act like the Authentic Self, and It doesn't think like the Authentic Self *ever* did.

Wait! You just realized that last sentence is very true. The Real You never talked or acted like this before... it wasn't until....

The Demon is a separate entity, and it is Not You who hates You. And for so long You have believed it *was* You that hated Yourself.

Say it again, say it with me if you like—Oh My God... the Demon isn't ME! It *isn't* really ME who's doing this!

"Alissa, I still don't get it...?"

The process of no longer equating your Self with your Demon will take time. The Demon has probably had months and/or years to tell you that you and It are one and the same. The revelation that the Real You is not It may hit you at first like a ton of bricks, but the work of untangling your Demon's talons from deep inside is not so immediate.

The more this idea begins to settle in your head, you may feel scared at times, because the Demon has taught you to believe in It and to give It your power. It's taught you to equate a self-destructive behavior with an identity. It's told you that you're no one without your binging, you'll never stop, you'll get *fat,* that you'll have no one else, and you have nothing else to excel at—and here comes Alissa to tell you the Real You was never the Demon to begin with. It can be a bit much at first; I know it was for me.

Your paradigms, or your ways of viewing the world and your place within it, are now just beginning to shift… this is the first step. Paradigm shifts are always a bit uncomfortable and nerve-wracking, but this time (unlike the Demon's try) I'm here to promise that this time, your new world view *will* be to your ultimate good.

After years of being kept powerless and confused, your Demon can feel how you're shifting something, that things are changing inside. It's getting worried… fearful even. It's hitting panic buttons in your head, making you feel like you need to throw this book across the room, to just run away and *keep* running away. But, you're not running away this time, are you? You've got a Flashlight, there's no need to keep running deeper into the darkness.

You can stop now, and face It instead. I'm right here with you.

What's the first action we take in fighting this? When I say give this Thing a name, I mean Give It a Name! Don't just call it an "eating disorder," Call It a Name! As you know, I call mine the Demon. I have heard others call it the Voice, the Inner Critic, Ana, Mia, Ed, my Evil Twin… personally, I'm fond of Fuckhead. You like Fuckhead? It pretty much describes what It's been doing inside you all this time, doesn't it?

Call It by a name, any name, that helps you continue to realize that the "eating disorder" and your Authentic Self are *not* one and the same entity.

What else can you do? Equally effective is the process of painting or drawing the Demon, giving it a face, and thereby giving It an externalized identity other than your own. You don't have to be an artist, just get some crayons or markers and remember back to when you were a child and drew pictures. If words are easier, remember that journal I spoke of? You can write descriptions of It, take the time to visualize this Thing. What does It look like? What images and colors do you associate with It, what emotions?

Want another idea? Many of us who suffer have gone online, thousands of websites and Myspace profiles glorify "Ana" and "Mia," praising their names as the vain attempt to appease the Demon long enough to be given a reprieve. The Demon is pleased to be set upon a pedestal, although It refuses to give pleasure in return, and never relents Its litany of demands due to the adulation. If you're one who has created a profile for your Demonized self already, consider starting a different one. Keep the old one if you wish, I know it can be hard to just let go of—besides, it can remind you of who your Demon wants you to be.

But create a new profile, make it as private as you wish, and let this profile reflect your Authentic Self. No thinspo. No dysfunctional words of self-recrimination and hatred. No numbers from the scale. Remember back to before the Demon took over, back to when you still had a life. Who were you long ago… back when things were still okay? Remember her… remember her often. We're going to talk more about her later.

These steps can help you to begin to pull this wretched creature off of you; once It is no longer You, You can confront It without confronting Yourself. As long as you continue to believe that the Real You is the one who is hurting herself, you're still under the Demon's influence, still operating under Its insidious lies. It is separate. It is not the Authentic Self.

It's not really You who is doing this to You.

Step back, peel It off of you and you can begin to look at It more objectively… It's just horribly hateful and ugly, isn't It? Why, It's uglier than you ever EVER were! And yet, instead of letting you see Its ugly face, It found a place to hide inside of you and told you that *you* were the ugly one, repeating that message until It made you a believer.

Remember, there is an Authentic Self.

The Real You is not lost for good, although you might fear she has been. The Real You has been shut inside a tiny, dark oubliette and left there, her voice replaced by the voice of the Demon, her loving heart ripped open and pierced by Its unforgiving claws.

Use your Flashlight, you can find her. She's waiting, and she knows you're beginning this fight. For the first time in so long, she knows there is Hope, a real Hope of breaking out of this cage that overtook her. She's cheering for you, can you hear her yet? She needs your help so badly, she's been waiting, locked in the darkness, alone for so long.

In the <u>Lord of the Rings</u> trilogy, the powerful magician Gandalf comes to meet with King Theoden of Rohan to seek his aid. When Gandalf arrives, the once-great King is failing; his health and vitality are slipping away as he lives under the influence of the evil wizard Saruman. Visions and illusions played in his head, with Grima Wormtongue there to whisper poisonous thoughts in King Theoden's ear… and the messages were relentlessly never-ending.

What images did King Theoden see while his mind was held trapped, his body wasting away from neglect? What promises were made to *him*, made and made… but never kept?

The King grew feeble under the influence of Saruman's black magic. He believed he was doing the right thing for his people, his kin, himself… but to all who loved him, they could see he was most obviously dying, daily becoming a mere shell of the man he once was. The evil magic was slowly draining him, never relenting. But, none of his kin or the nobles knew how to break the spell. They didn't know what to do to save him.

But, Gandalf knew. Gandalf wasn't fooled, not one bit, and Gandalf used his own intrepidity to get a weapon inside when weapons were forbidden (the Demon likes us defenseless). For Gandalf, his forbidden weapon was his magical staff.

This is the moment, this Flashlight, this book, is *your* magical staff. It is the Truth… and it's the one thing the Demon has tried to keep you from ever finding. Like Theoden's Demon, yours wants to keep you helpless while It sucks away your personal energy until the day you expire. But, I'm not going to let It keep up Its lies. See this knob? Turn the switch all the way; we're kicking it into High Beam.

Throw off the glamour! Throw off the evil magic of Saruman, the Demon who has captured and held you fixed. Realize that *It* was controlling you... that something Else, something Terrible, has been clouding your mind with lies and Hate and Fear.

The Real You never thought those horrific thoughts. The Real You never said those terrible things. The Real You is a creature of energy and light, and is inherently beautiful and perfect. Only the Demon tricked you into thinking you weren't. Embrace the glimmer of Hope you're feeling inside right now... it's *okay* to feel good. The Demon told you that you'd never feel good again, that's because It's lived on your Pain.

Remove the glamour that has shielded you from seeing the Truth, and then you will begin to breathe deeply once again. You will begin to see the world again, to laugh with real laughter in your heart. To feel real Joy. To know and feel Love, to give it and receive it freely once more.

These messages of Hatred that have been controlling you, manipulating you... they NEVER came from inside you! The Real You never used to think that way, or act that way. The Real You remembers the golden light of the sun, she remembers her innocent understanding of God, the Divine Source of Love, Light and Truth, and she wants so much to bathe in those warm rays once more.

The Hate? The hurt you're so used to feeling? Those emotions came from Saruman. They came from the Demon. They aren't really yours, they were given to you, thrust upon you daily until you accepted them as your own.

The Real You, like King Theoden, is waiting to awaken once more, to return to her place of power, her role of running the vehicle of your body and mind. The Demon took over the controls, and told you for so long that You Couldn't Do It Alone. That It was better at making decisions than you were. That you should allow It to take over.

And slowly, insidiously slowly... It did.

Let's go back now to where we started, the newscaster who told us of the women who were feeling "the pressure to look thin." Pressure? Oh baby, you ain't even begun to describe the Demon's oppressive sense of mental claustrophobia, pain and terror... but the "pressure to look thin" that we feel didn't come from an external source… it didn't come from images in a fashion magazine.

It came from the Demon. And…

The Demon… Isn't… ME!

✠Fighting the Demon✠

Alright, let's sit down and take a moment to rest, shall we? There's no sense charging straight into this thing head-on. After all, we've got some time to stop and try to figure it all out.

You feeling a little less shaky now? No, not yet? Well, that's alright. I'm not leaving you. I'm not giving up.

This Thing in Your Head… it's had a long time to teach you what It wants, and what It doesn't want you to think. Bet you don't know why? That's because in order for It to survive, It has needed your Hate. It grew larger each time you found a new avenue to spread Hate… Hate for yourself, Hate for your body, Hate for your past and your present, Hate and Hate and HATE!!!

Hate is exhausting though. It takes so much outta you to work up that much Hate and carry it around, every single day. And for years, you've been convinced that it's You who Hates You. Which feels terrible!

You know now that it was the Demon who hated you. You've stopped seeing the Demon as the same thing as yourself, which is the Demon's first loss of power and your first gain. You've given It a name, a name which will remind you that You are not It.

You know better now, my love. You're getting smarter than It, and It just *hates* that, huh? Well… let the Demon worry. It's about to start losing Its form, if you can stop feeding It.

"What, Alissa?"

That's right. Your Hate has kept this Demon strong; your negative emotions are the food source that It has lived off. Everything in the Universe needs an energy source to grow or to maintain form. Your Demon is no different.

Why else has this entity tried to foster only negative emotions in you? Why *doesn't* It allow you to feel good, to feel Loved? We'll explore that more in the next chapter. For now, let's give you some tools to start dealing with your Demon now that you know how to recognize It as being a separate (and disgusting) entity from yourself.

Ready? Okay, this is really the grand irony… you're gonna get off on this part once I tell ya, really. It's so sick and wonderful and twisted… wanna know how we fight the Demon after we've named It?

WE STARVE IT!

Now, didn't that make you smile?

I know it did. That's because of the grand irony in addressing these kinds of energetic problems… you get to turn the Demon's methods back on It! In fact, I'm going to teach you to start turning as many of the Demon's behaviors against It as I can.

Alright, to brass tacks… why and how do you starve a Demon? You starve a thought form to take away Its power. For an eating disorder, if you deprive It of the energy of the lower emotions which It came from and can only exist upon, then It cannot continue Its form of control and It begins to collapse.

Your Demon only exists on that which It inherently is… which is, essentially, Hate. It has sought to keep you, the host, in a state of perpetual Hate and Pain, in order to assist Its own growth. The more Hate you fed It, the bigger and bigger It got in your head—and that meant, over time, the more It could control how you saw things, could manipulate how you felt about them, and how you felt about yourself. It stole your words for help and then food from your own mouth, all in order to make Itself grow fat and happy on the Pain inside your head.

It gorged Itself on your mental anguish all this time while you've been starving and hurting! What a fuck, eh?

Grab your journal, or just a piece of paper. It's time we look at what this Demon has been up to inside you for so long.

On one side of the paper, you're gonna write out *everything* that the Voice has said to you thus far in your life. I know, your first thought is, "There's not enough paper… not in the entire world," but let's just try with one piece for now, trust me. List every accusation, every single Hate-filled message that your Demon has ever whispered in your inner ear.

Write the words, the exact words, that It likes to use. Write down every name It's ever called you, including the adjectives—"fat, disgusting, worthless pig," "fucking fatty," "pathetic, ugly cow." (Funny how many barnyard animals It comes up with when name-calling, isn't it? Mine always did anyhow.)

Write it out, and write more. Turn the paper over if you need to. Don't keep reading right now, get a paper and pencil and just scribble until the words begin to run dry. Then stop and take a look.

My GOD!

For one thing… no matter how many examples you came up with for your list, there aren't nearly as many as you thought there were gonna be, right? That's because, while in your head, the Demon has spun Its falsehoods into multitudinous and grandiose visions of failure and shame. When really, *this* is all It can come up with to say. And, it's a lot less than you ever expected to see. But, there it is.

And, another thing… this Demon, It hasn't come up with one original thought yet! The names and insults, they've grown so large and complicated in imagery as the Demon has grown inside your head. But, when you begin to take them out and examine them, my goodness! Look how quickly they almost all sound like the Exact Same Thing.

This, my love… this is why I can fight It. It never changes Its tune because It doesn't know how to. It says essentially the same thing to each and every one of us, finding the just-right mix of personal information that exists inside you to use as Its ammunition. It finds the most hurtful words and moments of your past, and reminds you of them constantly in order to reinforce Its message of Pain and shame. That is the Demon's *modus operandi*.

Why does It do this? So It can be strong by living off your Hatred.

Now… we've done the first half of this exercise, we've filled the left column with every single message we could think of. Label this side "The Demon," or you can use the name you've given It.

On the right side, label that as "Me," or my Authentic Self, or just use your own first name. And, start listening inside to the voice of your Authentic Self whom you've shut down and ignored for as long as you could without knowing why. She is the Authentic Voice which we have lost. Listen for her... she has suffered in silence long enough, only you can remove her gag.

Reread the Demon's messages, and then one by one, address them with the voice of your Authentic Self. If you wrote on the Demon's side: "You're always lazy, and selfish," consider that before filling in your own side. Was it really laziness that got you through school? Was it really selfish to try to eat a bagel, to feed your body?

Or was it a Lie?

The Demon's Lies control your mind in order to perpetuate your Pain, which It has needed to survive. YOU have never done anything to hurt yourself. YOU have never called yourself a single name. YOU still have Love to give, even to yourself. Yet, your body has suffered in direct correlation to the suffering the Demon causes you in your head.

The mind, body and spirit are intimately connected. We're gonna talk about healing all three, because all three must be addressed in order for you to cure yourself.

Let us not forget... this may be a Demon, but It wants to control your mind AND body by using your spirit. Your physical body needs your help, needs nourishment, just as much as your emotional self does. Even still, an eating disorder victim lives inside mental spheres where the ability to feed ourselves is terribly, TERRIBLY hard. It causes full scale Fear to even *think* about eating a meal... about the very idea of having to face the scale, or look in the mirror afterwards.

"But Alissa, you have no idea what I'll do to myself next if I let myself eat this," you cry in despair. Alissa is here to remind you... *you're* not doing anything to yourself. Your Demon is doing this. As long as It controls the puppet's strings, and keeps you hidden in the Lie that You and It are One and the Same, you cannot recover. Your Authentic Self remains caged.

Examine the process once more... the Demon creates Pain whenever we consider eating....

Think... *think*. Use your emotional intelligence and examine this with me. The Demon knows you need food to survive, as a human. It knows It needs your Fear and Hate for It to survive too. What an ideal, continual food source for the beast... It interjected the negative emotions that It needs (Fear and Hate) into something that *you* need for your own survival (Food). It basically built Its meals around your negative emotions about your meals.

That's so not fair! What the hell is that all about? Why should It get to eat, and you get to starve and/or throw up what little you put into yourself?

It's insidious, this Demon of ours. It's really one helluva sneaky bastard. It took me a goodly while to examine this shifty rat to discover Its true nature, but more and more, the Light of Truth is beginning to truly illuminate things for you, isn't it?

Go back to your paper again. Answer every message the Demon has told you with the Truth. Once you've answered It on paper, you've just practiced the next step—how to start answering It in your head.

Your next step will be to step onto the battlefield of your mind. On any given day, when the Demon starts up with Its tirade as usual, now you're gonna be more and more ready for the full frontal assault.

Your weapon is the Flashlight I've given you, your magical staff, the ability to see the Truth. It is the voice of your Authentic Self. Use your weapon often.

Let me show you how. Think back on some of the Rules and how your Demon never kept Its word, never let you feel better even when you followed Its every demand. But this time, talk back to It in your head.

The Demon said: *If you eat under 800 calories today, and do 200 crunches before bed, you won't be so repulsive to look at... I'll let you feel a little bit better.*

The Real You said: I did eat under 800 calories, and did *400* crunches… and I still feel miserable. You lied to me, Demon.

The Demon said: *You're alone in this, and no one is ever going to help you, or understand you, or even LIKE you, because you're so disgusting and pathetic.*

The Real You said: You liar, it was *you* who taught me to be disgusting. You told me so for long enough that I actually fell for it. I believed your lies, Demon. You taught me to keep everyone away, to let no one in. You made me isolated and lonely, first in my head and then in my real life, and then you taught me how to hurt myself while you grew fat on my Pain.

This is exactly how you begin the war, with the onslaught of the truth, spoken by the Authentic Self. First, you must learn to recognize the disorder as being separate from the Real You. Then, you must learn to tell yourself the Truth, in spite of the Demon's messages—do it on paper first, and then, start doing it in your head.

What else can help you in this fight, right here and now? Breaking the isolation; it's another important step in reclaiming your Authentic Self from the Demon's grasp. When It tells you that you are alone, list the people in your life who Love you. Look at the network around you, right now… in your very own life, even it's just one other person… think on how they feel about you. How would they describe you? And, if you stopped denying their compliments, how would you really feel about the words they use to describe you? How different are those words from your Demon's? Night and day kinda different, huh?

The more we begin to seek, the more answers begin to appear.

You see, once you get these things outside your head and into words on paper, you're making It concrete. You're turning It into something that can't keep hiding, can't keep up the masquerade as the Authentic Self. It's *not* You. The more you look at this thing, the more it makes sense.

Fight the Demon with your Authentic Voice. Fight the Demon with your words of defiance against It; think the words that you say to It in your head, or say them aloud if you're in a situation that allows you to literally Speak Up. Use the growing sense of strength inside that the

Light is helping you to nourish, and be courageous! You already know how to Hate, your Demon taught you well. Now use the Demon's methods against It, learn to focus your rage against It instead of against your body and yourself.

In the coming days, even after you've written out the Demon's messages—even if you've listed them several times on several different days because repetition and practice with talking back is helpful—you're gonna keep hearing the same old shit in your head. The Demon never gets new tapes, just makes up variations on the same old ones.

"But, Alissa... does that mean I have to have an ongoing Demon dialogue in my head for the rest of my life, just to get Healthy again?"

Nahhhhh. Don't let your Demon pull any tricks on ya. The Truth is... wait, I'll turn up the Flashlight a little more....

As you begin to confront It, It will begin to shrink. As the Demon begins to lose Its form, It begins to lose Its behavioral domination over the host. You are literally starving It to death when you learn how to stop the ongoing cycle of Hate.

The first step is recognizing It as something very separate from the Real You.

Next, learning to confront It begins to dissolve the iron-grip It's had on your willpower, and your continued obedience to Its Rules. When the Rules begin to crumble, they become easier to let go of, and *then* the magic occurs.

Imagine a world with no Rules. No scales. No judgment. No Pain. It's real... and it's waiting for you.

When we make room in our lives by removing one thing, there is space for something new and beautiful to grow in its place—this is as applicable to the Demon as it is rearranging furniture or weeding a garden. And this will take time. You must be patient with yourself during the process. It took time for all this mental crap to build up inside, it will take time for you to remove it all.

Stinky ottomans in your head? Time to get rid of some of that old baggage. And as you discard it, look at all the room you have now for Hope. For growth. For starting anew.

Let me repeat this, the more you continue to exorcise the Demon's messages, the more It slowly shrinks. In time, It begins to lose Its form. Why? Because It's not getting as much energy as It's used to. The source of hatred within you is changing, and It cannot bear the change (anything containing the essence of Love is unbearable to a Demon).

Therefore…

It shrinks in the amount of space It occupies in your head, so you can hear your Authentic Voice more and more often.

It shrinks in Its ability to coerce your emotions and world view, convincing you with half-thoughts of loneliness, isolation, and your own innate despair, your disgust with your body and your life.

And It shrinks in Its ability to control your physical actions; the starving, the binging, these changes are the last thing It lets go of as It grows feeble and weak in the presence of Love.

As you shift the hatred away from yourself and onto It, It loses Its dominion over you.

Your self-rage can begin to melt away when the fighting against yourself ceases inside, and becomes instead the fight against the Demon. Gradually, It is forced to let go of Its ability to manipulate your emotions to Its insidious, Pain-creating ends, and later, without negative emotions to perpetuate your self-destructive actions, the behaviors are easier to resist. The episodes of starving, or purging, grow fewer and further apart as It shrinks and shrinks like Shrinky Dinks.

The more you continually confront Its lies and starve It, the shorter the Demon's messages will get—"You're still fat!" But the Demon's lies become like weak blows after having been under the lash for so very long. The more you practice fighting It, the easier It gets to fight against. But it does take time, so you must be patient when the changes don't come all in a day, or a week, or a month.

From now on, you must be on guard. Be wary; now, you are wiser about the true nature of It than It *ever* wanted you to be, and that's to your ultimate advantage. You must be ready to catch the thought the minute the Demon presents it. It takes a little practice, but you're gonna get better at it. Haven't you always succeeded in absolutely everything else you really put your mind to? Well, why should this be different, especially when you know how much you honestly *do* want to Love again?

Let's practice…

You're not really going to eat that, you disgusting pig, are you?

I am, I'm gonna eat this toast *and* the banana next to it. And, You can't stop me. Oooh and look, I'm using butter again. What do you think of that, asshole?

You'll get fat. Go throw it right back up, you worthless whore before you blimp out.

No, you can't make me do that, only I can. You can make me *think* about throwing up, and you can even try to create enough Fear inside to enact your awful wish. But, YOU can't make me. Only I make me… and You're not ME.

You are growing in strength and wisdom now, you are the fighter-in-training no longer… the battle field is yours, and you will slowly gain back lost ground if you continue the fight against the Enemy. The more you turn Its messages of shame and hate against It, answering those accusations and lies with words of Love and Truth, the more the Demon knows It can't get to you. You will get stronger, and It will grow weaker.

It's like Teflon, baby… the crap your Demon keeps slinging each day? It starts to slide right off. Gotta build up your shield though. Gotta practice talking back, practice getting your Voice back. And, I'll say it again, it takes time; it doesn't happen in a day. It takes *time,* so be patient with yourself if you have some "bad" days, or weeks or whatever, along the way.

Perhaps, you don't believe me yet? You don't believe there's hope that your mind can ever make this change, much less your body ever accept food inside it the way I'm talking about. You're certain you're too far gone; the Demon has had too long inside to twist you to Its Pain.

It's okay, my dearest. Hold my hand, I told you… sometimes we need to stop and rest along the way. The Light takes a while to get used to—it took me months and months to get used to it. It's like putting food back in your stomach, at first the sensation may feel a little… odd. Scary. Uncomfortable. You can only handle so much, but you know how much you want and need more. And just like food, slowly you're gonna get used to it, especially as your mind and body begin to react to the nourishment you're finally providing after spending so long in deprivation.

It's *okay* to love yourself. Your Demon told you how unworthy you were, but now you know It's a lying bastard. Close your eyes, right now, and give yourself a hug inside your heart. If tears come, let them flow… the water from your eyes will melt the stone that's replaced your heart.

"Alissa, I can't. I just can't. I see nothing inside, I feel nothing…."

I'm going to teach you another trick to help you, some mental judo to get you through the blockages. Your Demon has twisted your perception of reality, correct? You know that, of course you do—your perception of your body didn't match anyone else's while this Demon's been running things, the girl in the mirror looked fatter every day to nobody but *you*. And until lately, you've only had the Demon to listen to, so you didn't know why your sense of perception was so out of whack with what others saw.

Well, now you're going to use the power It taught you to twist your perception of reality to your own advantage.

As the Demon's messages continue, and they do continue on for a while before the blather ever stops, but until it does… each time the Demon tells you a message of Hate, stop.

Halt!

Replace in your mind the image of the child that you were. Before you were broken by the Demon. When you still knew how to give Love and receive it. When you could still feel Joy. That child is in you. That beautiful, lovely child is your Authentic Self. See her hair in the sunlight and how it would feel to your touch, gaze into her eyes and watch her smile. Make her real inside you.

Imagine now that you're the caretaker of this exquisite child. When the Demon tries to speak, examine Its words as if they were being addressed directly to her. Would you speak to a child with such berating words of shame and hate as the Demon tries to do? Would you deny this beautiful, innocent girl the food her body needs, just to be mean to her and to punish her for imagined wrongdoings? Just to test her willpower? Would you force her to throw it up as soon as she was done?

You wouldn't dare. If you were *that* kind of person, then the Demon we have? It wouldn't have manifested as an eating disorder. Your heart is like mine, and like all our sisters and brothers out there... it's been broken by the Demon's lies, but it knows how to Love. It knows what real Love feels like, your heart remembers.

You would hold that little angel in your arms, and tell her what a precious gift she is, and how much she has to offer this world, how much she will learn. You would encourage her to reach towards others if she was hurting, instead of teaching her to keep those who love her distant and impossible to reach like the Demon demands. You would teach her to love the food she ate, to enjoy the act of eating and to glory in the many tastes, as well as the contented sensation of a full belly.

You would Love her.

Answer the Demon, and turn this new perception upon It. Let your ability to twist reality begin to work towards your freedom, instead of your ongoing imprisonment. It will take practice, but everything does. Be patient, and keep believing.

You're so fat and ugly, I can't stand to look at you in the mirror.

Stop....

Picture the child.

See her innocent eyes, her trusting face.

Would you let this Demon talk to her that way? Or would you protect her and fight for her until the day she is strong enough to protect herself? She's not ready yet, so it's up to you. Tell that bastard off until the day she is ready to take over.

…These are beautiful hands you have. They have so much more to be doing, so many good things to complete in this world, if they could be retrained to do what always came naturally… until the Demon took control.

At one point, while in the midst of my months-long mental recovery process from my eating disorder, I realized something powerful. It stopped me in my tracks, literally, as I was walking back to work from lunch one day.

The Golden Rule… Do Unto Others as You Would Have Them Do Unto You.

"Yeah, yeah, Alissa. Heard it."

But… wait. The thing I always stumbled on… it was right there in front of me. I could treat *others* so much better than I could ever begin to treat *myself* with this Demon calling the shots.

Now, I had to treat *myself* like I would treat *others*.

I was nice to everyone else in the world, but one person. I would never use my Demon's language of hatred when talking to or about another person, only when talking about *me*. Now, if I really wanted to get better, I had to learn to be nice… to me.

I had never considered how much I had lived on the opposite end of the equation… giving and giving, and never even considering something so "selfish" as giving back to myself. My Demon had taught me that was wrong, and I had believed It.

But, I was getting wiser. And, so are you. See? You're not squinting so much now as when we first began. The Light gets easier along the way, doesn't it?

Consider this… there is a card in the Tarot deck called "The Devil." The Waite-Colman-Smith illustration shows a fearsome, horned Demon with a man and a woman standing before him. Each naked and completely vulnerable person wears huge, loose-fitting shackles about their necks, and the chains of these shackles lead straight back to the Demon. In a reading, the card tells us we are in the presence of the Great Liar… that we have been deceived or, worse yet, we are deceiving ourselves.

The shackles that bind these people to the Demon could easily slip over their heads; they could set themselves free at any time. *But they chose not to.* The Demon presents the self-destructive behaviors, and we willingly put the shackle on ourselves… binding ourselves to the lies of a drug addiction, alcoholism… or an eating disorder. Because we were tricked by the Great Liar.

It is not the last card in the Major Arcana, the Devil is not the end of the road. He only feels like it, because there we are… stuck in our chains that we put on, all by ourselves, and staying right there with the one who Lies to us, believing that in doing so… we're still living. We're managing, we're coping… we're making it by. Day by day.

And inside, the Authentic Self grieves, and waits, and hopes for the day when the shackle is finally discarded.

Look at the shackle you've put on your neck. See how it has kept you chained to this Beast? It is easy for you to remove, and yet… it isn't. Like Bilbo having to give up the Ring of Doom in the <u>Lord of the Rings</u> trilogy. He pines for it, even as he knows it is time to let it go. It has had a long time to work its evil magic on his soul. He hates it, he loves it. He can't imagine life without it, and yet he knows in order to live, he must find a way to let it go.

A part of you loves being disordered. Your Demon let you fall in love with It and no one else. But even your Demon knows you could leave any time, that if you fell in love with yourself again, you would leave. So

It lies and lies, and keeps you right there in Its evil grasp for as long as It can, possibly forever. Hating yourself, loving It.

I wish I could say it's a straight path back, it's not. Bad days will still happen, at any step along your path… and that's okay too. It feels very strange to distance yourself from a paradigm, an established thought pattern that you've lived with for so long. You may feel yourself disconcerted, kinda of two minds for awhile, as the battlefield changes inside your head.

But, when we address the cause, the symptoms will follow. So many other eating disorder resources and programs focus solely on the sufferer's symptoms (starving, binging, purging, low self esteem, depression) never realizing they are pulling the weed from the topsoil yet leaving the root behind.

Mind, body and spirit. It takes all three.

The Demon is the cause; It infected all three aspects within you. But You are not It. You are the caretaker of the Authentic Self, the golden child kept safe inside.

Use these tricks to begin finding your Authentic Voice, your Authentic Self—the fight *does* get easier over time. Answering the Demon's messages with words of Love and Protection… that takes practice, so practice often, okay?

The hardest part you've already done… you reached out. The Demon told you that you couldn't and yet, you're reading this… right now. You are already beating It, and the war will get easier as you gain confidence in the arena.

For years you listened and simply Obeyed. Now, you can begin to take your power back. A bite at a time.

You are Not Helpless against It.

❧Thought forms☙

"How did you get this Demon anyhow? Is it abuse related? Is it the pressure to look a certain way? Was it your parents, was it your dancing? Was it something I said or did; is this *my* fault?"

These are the questions that the non-afflicted ask us. They cannot even begin to fathom how such a horrible state of mind can come to be in someone they love so much. And, most terribly, we are unable to give them any answers—we also don't know what or why. We can't even begin to talk about It, much less understand It.

This is when the Light is going to get slowly brighter and brighter. We'll begin with the brightest Source there is… Spiritual, or Universal law. The concepts of these laws may seem unusual at first, and I encourage you to take the time you need to consider them as you read. The ideas themselves are not new or original, they are not uniquely mine, but are often described by the world's mystical religions as well as many modern metaphysical resources.

The term I use, "the Source," is another way to describe Divinity, or God. I visualize the Source as meaning That from which we came and which we seek to evolve towards. The Source is supremely benevolent and abundant; lacking in judgment and endlessly compassionate, the Source is that which we find within ourselves during our best moments when living a material life. There is a Hindu saying which reminds us of our innate Divinity, "Thou are That."

Our emotions are like odometers which measure our proximity to the Source, an ongoing feedback mechanism meant to motivate ourselves into any necessary changes when we've grown too distant from God.

Emotions are the key. Emotions are what got you here to this hell, what keep you here in hell, and what can set you free. For a long time, you've taught yourself to ignore your bad emotions, to stuff away the rage and pain without ever daring to examine *why* you chose to stay so far from the Source. And living in the absence of any Love or Light became a terribly normal state of being. Why?

(Because Demons don't come from the Source, and It hates the Source with all Its might, and so It has instilled the same values in you… but let's not jump too far ahead yet).

Let's first talk about how you understand yourself.

We are intimately familiar with perceiving the notion of our Self as being part material, that is our bodies, and part non-material, that is, our minds… our emotions, thoughts and feelings. But, this is not all we are made of.

We are energetic beings. We emit energy and we absorb it. Christians call this energetic body the "soul." In Hinduism, the term "prana" refers to the life energy within; in Chinese philosophy, they call it "chi." Our emotions can be visualized as a prismatic display of this personal energy, and like light and sound waves, emotions also travel at low levels that vibrate slowly, and at high levels with a fast vibration.

The closer we align ourselves to the Source, the faster our emotions vibrate. We become brighter. And to find out where you're at right now, start examining your emotions. They are the roadmap only you can use to navigate your own course, from within.

To reiterate this… emotions are expressions of personal energy. The image of the prism which separates white light into many colors symbolizes the way in which we separate our energy into our emotions. If an emotional descriptive could be given to the Source itself, I like to think we'd call it "Bliss." The higher attuned we are to the Source, the more we align ourselves to That Which We Truly Are, and this is felt by the higher emotions of Love, Generosity, Kindness, and Compassion.

The low levels of emotional energy encompass the lower emotions, those of Hate, Fear, Guilt, Depression, Rage and Shame. The closer our emotions travel to the ultimate Source, the lighter and higher our personal vibratory frequency becomes. Hope, Joy, Charity, Happiness… all of these emotions are closer to the Source.

But when we remain in the lower realms for an extended time as a human, it can be terribly easy to get stuck there.

Energy, prana, follows its own set of inherent Universal laws. The subjects of Universal (or Divine) Law as well as thought forms, have been broached by various religions for centuries, as well as the metaphysical community at large, and books on both subjects are already in existence. Books by Wayne W. Dyer superlatively describe the Source, and how aligning one's self with Universal Intention can create miracles in one's life; Tibetan theosophy describes *tulpas,* or materialized thoughts which do the creator's bidding. I encourage you, if the idea tickles your fancy, to read more on the subject of Universal Law and thought forms by other authors. Knowledge is Power.

Suffice to say, I am not the first to propose these concepts, but I *am* the first to tell you that the Demon whose been eating you alive is really a thought form.

And, guess who created It?

You did.

"But… wait a minute. What's a 'thought form?'"

Every moment that we are thinking, we are creating thought forms. We are… right now as you read this… creating among us, a new thought form. This book is the external materialization of a thought form I had… that of my desire to use my wisdom and my words to publish a book that would help others recognize and thereby combat the Demon.

The brand new, fragile emotion inside called Hope that you're just beginning to allow yourself to feel? It needs fed. It's a brand new thought form, and It came from the Light. Keep believing in yourself and you'll keep feeding It while I try to explain.

A thought form is made by us from the energy of our thoughts. There is a Rosicrucian saying which I have adopted as a personal business motto, "Thoughts are things and words have wings."

Thoughts are things. They take form. These forms materialize on the mental, or creative, plane. Can you see this plane? No, it is immaterial; however, do not mistake immateriality for inconsequentiality. Just as our bodies inhabit the material plane, our thoughts inhabit the mental plane, which overlaps (or co-exists) with the material realm. Just as you realize your Self as being part body and part mind, you are also part energy and exist in all these planes, at all of these levels, simultaneously.

In the study of the Qabalah, our human existence is imagined as being of several different planes; the author Lon Milo DuQuette likens these planes to the floors of a metaphysical building, which stands as the metaphor of our lives. He describes at the bottom floor is the material realm, and above it stands a formative plane, and a creative plane. Inhabiting these realms are creatures of our own making; angels, as he calls them, which are created by our thoughts, which stem from our emotions.

And in the same floor where the Angels play, the Demons can also lie in wait. Even still, the power of these creatures does not come from them… it comes from us; the information from the top floor, or your highest angels, acts as the built-in, trickle-down method of inspiration which becomes the material actions that shapes the destiny of our lives. It is a dance of that which you continually create, that which you maintain, and that which you destroy, as the dancing Hindu god Lord Nataraja reminds us.

Every one of us, from a child at play, to an adult arguing with her boss, is creating a thought form. Thought forms are made with the amount of personal energy, that is, the quality and amount of emotional energy, we put into the thought. Ever heard the saying, "an idea that built up steam?" That's the exact image. It grows and takes Its form as It is thought of repeatedly, feeding and increasing It until the thought form begins to interact more concretely with the material plane.

Some thoughts are less cohesive than others. The scattered thoughts and the to-do lists of our normal days do not contain much of our personal energy or emotion. That is, we create the thought form at the moment the idea comes to us, we complete it, and the energy is expended. If I think about picking my son up in a few hours, and in a few hours from now, I've completed the task, normally I wouldn't reflect on the passing thought of a few hours back ever again. The thought form contained little emotion, it has expended itself, and I am not giving it more energy in order to assist it in growing.

"How do you 'give energy' to a thought form? You just said they're immaterial."

Our emotions emanate as expressions of our personal energy and are dynamic and changing—the better the mood we're in, the "higher" our vibratory signal we currently emit. Thought forms can be visualized as a coalescence of emotions, which can only take in more of the same emotion in order to gain shape and potency.

What is the nature of such a thing? A thought form is what it is at the moment we create one… and, unlike more advanced beings such as ourselves, *they cannot develop or evolve beyond that of their original intention at the time of creation*. That is, they contain the emotion and intention of the Creator (us) and cannot change their nature, as set at the moment of intention (by us).

Intention is everything. I want you to remember that. We'll touch back on it often.

With our emotional intentions, we can create positive and negative thought forms. A positive thought form enhances our path towards the higher emotions; a negative thought form inhibits that path, dragging our emotions down. Our actions reflect our emotional impulses; when filled with joy, our actions are also filled with joy. When filled with sorrow, not only our thoughts, but our actions increase our sorrow. Like attracts like… Love attracts Love, and Pain attracts Pain.

A Demon, your eating disorder, came from a moment of Pain, and It can only know more Pain in order to grow strong and continue to dominate the actions of Its host… you.

So, how *does* a negative thought form come to dominate a personality? How do you know if such a thing is even happening? I'll tell you how. They leave calling cards. Those calling cards manifest as self-destructive behaviors enacted by the human host.

As a thought form, It understands the power that emanates from us, the Creator. Like all forms, It too wants to grow, It is hungry… and the thoughts of Pain are delicious. Demons can only take in more of that which They are; a thought form born of Pain needs more Pain in order to increase Itself.

Therefore, It seeks to create an emotional state of perpetual Pain, and to use Its power in the mental realm to manipulate the host's emotions and thereby manifests as self-destructive behavioral patterns in the material realm—this behavior can be an eating disorder, but it can also be alcoholism, drug dependency, cutting and many other lifelong, destructive behavioral patterns. My specialty, my Demon's forte, was anorexia and bulimia, which is why I touch on those behavior patterns most often for this work.

Thought forms are not the enemy. If anyone is, it's us. We must think the thoughts to create the Pain to help It to grow. Only *we* can think what we think... but, negative thought forms, Demons, are tricksters. The Demon teaches us how to make ourselves our own Worst Enemy, and then hides Its true nature by masquerading as our very own thoughts.

But, remember what we already know of It?

The Demon... Isn't... ME!

I repeat, not all thought forms are malevolent or should be feared. They are not the enemy, in and of themselves. Intention is *everything* and only the Creator sets the intention. We do.

"Gods, archangels, angels, spirits, intelligences, and demons are personifications of all our abilities and potential abilities—a wondrous hierarchy of consciousness that represents the subdivision of our own soul," writes Lon Milo Duquette.[1]

Let's look at one non-threatening thought form that many of us *have* experienced. Infatuation... falling in love. When we fall in love, we are feeling emotions of the highest frequencies and generating extremely high levels of energy... we are creating a thought form: the thought of

---

[1] DuQuette, Lon Milo. The Chicken Qabalah of Rabbi Lamed Ben Clifford (York Beach, ME: Weiser Books, Inc. 2001) p.134.

our Beloved and the positive feelings of union that are found when we are with them.

We feed this form with the emotional energy It requires, that which It was born from. To grow, It needs a state of perpetual Love in the host, and seeks to create this. And so, as we first become smitten, we find ourselves thinking on the person repeatedly, thoughts of Love. Thoughts that are created from our higher emotions, and are therefore of a higher energetic frequency.

Sometimes, our first fall is followed by an immediate crush... the person we were so smitten with never called. The thought form is no longer being fed; It's no longer being repetitively considered, nor given the host's emotional energy. Like a crush, you can remember how it took your heart a little time to let go, but you did... the emotions of Love weren't there to sustain that thought form any longer. And new thought forms have come in to replace the space left by the old.

Then, there are the happier times when the one with whom we've given our heart is returning our intentions. The Beloved's emotions are now generating even *more* emotions within us for the thought form to exist upon, and the quality of these emotions is much more powerful than the glancing thoughts we give other personages in our daily lives. We think long and often about the one we Love, we think about being together again soon... when you saw him last, and when you'll see him again. What he said, and then what you said, and how he kissed you, and what his lips felt like when he did.

We feed the thought form with our rapturous emotions and pleasurable mental expenditure. It grows larger and larger inside us, and we are happy to have It "drive the vehicle" of the human host every now and then; the world seems to sparkle it is so full of wonder, and we are prone to daydreaming. That is, the thought form is creating an emotional and mental state in the host which perpetuates and feeds It Love, because It came from Love.

Notice first... the behaviors evidenced by this thought form are *not* self-destructive. This is your first indication that the thought form at play was created by the higher emotions. Because a thought form wants to become more, it continues to attract emotions of the same frequency, the same emotion that its Creator dictated at the point of origination. Therefore, as it gains in size and form, it fosters behaviors in the host that will continue to attract more Love, more Joy, more Bliss.

Higher frequency emotions are the ones that assist our souls as we continue to grow and evolve closer to the form of the Divine. When we are lost in a movie, or taken with the rapturous sounds of a symphony, we are in the midst of a high frequency emotion. It generates a buzz and energy inside that is lighter, more buoyant in nature, the signature of the Source.

These types of thought forms do not hate the Light. They do not fear discovery, and they do not seek to hide the Truth of their nature, ever. They are closer to the Source. The Divine Light, which can be envisioned as pure white, is the ultimate vibratory level that we all seek to know while traveling our soul's path. It is described by many mortal men as "the search for God," and in the seeking, we become more like God. Energetically, this is reflected by our vibrational signature which begins to attune itself to the Source's as we grow closer to God in our hearts, our minds and our physical actions. Universal law states it is our inherent nature to reach towards the Source in any given lifetime, unless another force acts upon the soul.

That Universal Law kinda sounds like regular ole physics, doesn't it? A force in motion will stay in motion, unless another force acts upon it. Our soul will continue to seek its upwards evolution towards the Source, unless we encounter another force that acts upon it... such as a malignant thought form. A Demon.

Thought forms that come from the higher frequencies are much less likely to attempt to permanently take over the host, to my own metaphysical understanding. Perhaps when a person becomes Enlightened, in the terms of the Masters, a mutual collaboration between host and thought form is made, allowing a very high frequency form to take over the vehicle of the host's body and mind in order to work towards creating even more Love, more Joy, for the host and for all of us. But I can only surmise as much.

And yet, not all thought forms are so benign as infatuation, are they? The one we know best, our Demon? It wasn't formed from these higher emotions at all. It preaches what It knows, and all It knows is what It came from, the lower emotions... It only knows how to Hate. Hate is what It attracts, because as we said, Like Attracts Like is another Universal Law.

Again, the evidence of self-destructive behaviors in someone's life are the calling cards of a malignant thought form that has now gained enough strength to begin attempting to "take over the vehicle," that is, the mind and body of the Creator, the host. The higher floors are dictating the movement on the bottom floor, the material realm—we complete the physical acts of starving and binging due to the hurtful emotional impulses inside, driven by our desperate thoughts.

A compulsion is a malignant thought form trying to "run the vehicle." An addiction is a malignant thought form that has begun the process of taking over Its host, ultimately often to Its own detriment, since thought forms take themselves out by taking out their host—be this by suicide, overdose, starvation, and/or acute cardiac arrest.

Demons aren't logical, but we'll use that knowledge to our advantage more later.

An eating disorder is another type of thought form that's trying to run the vehicle. But realistically It can't, that's why It speaks in such simple languages inside your head—think back about what the Demon actually says when we wrote it out. It's always the same old thing all the time, right? Right. The same names, the same insults, the same demands, the same forms of physical punishment.

It's not an advanced being. A thought form cannot advance beyond Its original intent at the time of creation.

Rage, Hate, Fear, Guilt, Pain. These emotions are *not* what our souls are innately composed of, nor what we are evolving towards, on a primary energetic level. They are (for most humans) very uncomfortable emotions to experience; we simply don't like feeling these ways. We usually don't like it so much, we'll find a way to stop feeling these things, thus pushing us towards experiencing the higher emotions instead, and moving us closer to the Source once more... a kind of built-in evolutionary model for our souls to keep us heading in the right direction.

And what about when those negative feelings simply *can't* be stopped? Bring on the anesthetics! Drugs, alcohol, sex, prescriptions, food, and control through starvation, numbness through binging... more more more!

Please God, I'm only human. I can't keep feeling this way, I've got to find a way to get away from it, to get Numb again, just to feel Good about myself, even if only for a little while.

But with a Demon in control, we can't even imagine allowing ourselves to feel *good*. The best we pray for is numbness... non-feeling. The best emotion a Demon can promise us is the ability to feel *no* emotion... which is to say, the Demon likes to take away your emotional compass. If your emotions tell you your proximity to the Source, feeling nothing gives you nothing to complain about (for the moment, it only takes the Demon a short while before the harassment returns full force for more Hate-making so It can eat).

The human condition is Hard. It's really, really hard down here, and it's really easy to lose our path, our direction. Our way towards the Light. In fact, that's kinda the point in incarnating anyhow. The Hindu term "lila" means the Divine Play, the game of life. Which path will you choose in this incarnation, your soul poses to itself... one of joy which advances your path to the Source, or one of Pain, which distracts you from your true purpose and delivers only devastation and heartache? And what will you ultimately learn and gain from this entire experience?

Each day we get up and roll the dice. Each day we have a new chance for a "do-over," a moment to realign ourselves, a chance to get just a little bit better. Each miniscule realignment, inch by inch, towards the Source adds up over time, and every day, a little more can be done.

It really *can* be done, and you're learning how, right now. You are already on that path, and your emotions will continue to give you the feedback you need on your soul's progress.

"What does it take to become vulnerable to such a hideous phenomenon? Do you have to be abused, or what? Is it because you were a dancer, and dancers have eating disorders?"

It takes emotions of the same origin to create a Demon, remember?

Any time we find ourselves in a deep, dark emotional place where we choose to stay, we are at risk. There is no easy equation as to who gets an eating disorder and who among us dodges the bullet. Not every victim of abuse later turns into an anorexic, not every anorexic was abused in her past. But, one thing is certain... a victim of abuse was strongly emitting at one point in her life a very low emotional frequency, one of Hate, Shame, Guilt, Pain, Depression.

She created a thought form born of this emotion and, for the Form to take over, she fell into the Demon's trap, willfully putting on the shackles and chains we discussed in the last chapter as It presented them, one by one. She gave it more Pain, and refused to resolve the real issue, but allowed it to malinger and fester. By turning her eyes from the true Source of her hatred, depression and shame, she gave the Demon a place to grow. And so It began the long and terrible masquerade as the Authentic Self... until now.

No matter who you are... right now... you need to begin to let it go. Whatever it was that started it all, let it go. You can't change what's already happened. You can't exorcise this Demon out of your mouth by purging until your throat is trashed. You can't prove your control over what happened by starving until your ribs are sore. The only way to conquer this is to truly be strong, take a deep breath, and admit to yourself it all began with Hate. You began to Hate yourself, and there was a catalyst, there was a reason why.

Think about when it first started, give yourself a moment to reflect back.... It's okay just to think about it. Remember, now isn't then, and you're only thinking about it. You're not reliving it, and you never will....

Look at the event that triggered it all, only you know what it is. Observe it as part of what will never happen in your life again. Realize you are *already* not the person you were when it happened. You have already changed. Your life has already changed. Your Demon gave you the idea that to keep strong, you had to suffer, you had to be *thin*. The Demon lied. Time passed, as it will always will... and you are never going to relive the hell that you went through then.

And you don't have to keep living in one now either.

Forgive yourself for once being weak. Forgive yourself for once being naïve. Forgive yourself for getting hurt. Forgive yourself completely. When you can truly forgive yourself, you can let go of the need to punish yourself.

Breathe. Breathe deeply while we take a moment to consider our sisters and brothers who have suffered, some unto death, from the Demon's demands we already know so well.

Anorexia, bulimia and fashion modeling seem to go together immediately in many people's minds – some might even know about Ana Carolina Reston, a Brazilian model who died at the age of 21 while following a tomato and apple diet that her Demon thought would suit her well. Demons aren't logical; hers went down with the ship when her physical body could no longer comply with the Hoops she was made to jump through every day, undoubtedly trying to keep the Demon's name-calling at bay as her profession doubled the pressure to maintain her emaciated look. Eventually, she escaped… but only in the most horrible way.

In the same year, after three months of a diet of lettuce leaves and Diet Coke, Luisel Ramos died on the catwalk at the ripe old age of 21 as well, following her younger sister who was also a model and died of anorexia at the age of 18. They didn't have a chance to "grow out of it" like some think we will do. For so many, the body reaches a terrible point of no turning back, and whether they intended to check out of this realm or not no longer matters. Or maybe, if we could have asked them, they would have told us they'd rather die than keep up with the pain of hating themselves, unaware they believed the Demon's Greatest Lie… that You and It are One and the Same… never knowing the Demon only masquerades as the Self, that It is something separate. The glamour never lifted; Gandalf never showed… no escape, no escape.

Why dancers, some may ask? The Demonic battle Gelsey Kirkland fought is famous, and some might know of the anorexia-induced death of Boston Ballet's Heidi Gunther… but even the non-professionals suffer. I should know–I was one of many I knew in my town alone. I danced as a child then left ballet during my teenage years, only to return to it again in college. After college, I began dancing and performing with our state's ballet companies and was often submerged ten or fifteen hours a week inside the dance studio in my mid-twenties, in the evenings after my full-time job. I slept, breathed, worked and danced.

Much like models, the mindset of a dancer creates a set of ideal conditions for an eating disorder. Dancers already demand perfection of themselves, the technique of ballet has a built-in system of extremely high expectations, and the atmosphere in so many studios is one of competition, which can easily lead to self-berating moments of frustration and rage, creating a fertile soil for the Demon's seed. We push ourselves harder, trying to dance better than the girl in the front row who's always the best. And if we *are* that girl in the front row, we have to work even harder to keep it up, to maintain.

The frustration with a bad day in the studio can so easily morph into the messages of the Demon, "You lazy fat cow, you can't even jump, jump higher!" We blame ourselves for our own deficiencies and we ask more of our bodies than most people do. Despite the demands we make, we are extremely hard on our body's physical difficulties, its injuries and complaints are routinely ignored in order to get the job done. And, after all, ignoring hunger is just learning to ignore a different kind of physical complaint.

Dancers are not the only type of athletes who use the technique of their art or sport in order to pursue such difficult goals of "perfection." Figure skaters and gymnasts often suffer from eating disorders – names like Christy Henrich, Erica Stokes and Kristie Phillips who admit to doing battle with the Demon. They are much like their sisters, the ballerinas. Professional body builders, actresses and stage performers. Mary-Kate Olsen, Ashlee Simpson, Tracey Gold, Sally Field, Paula Abdul… just a few who have had the courage to admit to their Demons' pain. Princess Diana of Wales… perhaps the most famous bulimic of our time. But what about those who don't admit it, those who are still obeying Rule Number One?

There are many faces with similar personality traits, all suffering, and all feeling so terribly alone. Feeling out of control, desperate to maintain order through a set of rigid definitions of what "perfect" will look like, what it will weigh, the right number on the scale.

And what about the boys? Jockeys, wrestlers, rowers, swimmers... all facing weight restrictions. All willing to go to desperate lengths to chase the Demon's image of perpetual perfection.

But, it doesn't take a model or an athlete to create a Demon. Any time we find ourselves in a prolonged state of despair, we are creating a potently negative thought form around us that will *never* evolve into a higher emotion. By staying grounded in this negative emotion, we open ourselves, and help It to grow stronger. It sucks on our newly-ripped emotional wounds, *whatever* it was that caused them, and spits poison into the open flesh while pretending to be "helping" you deal with that Pain by teaching you to Hate yourself and to hurt yourself.

There are thousands of reasons to explain why this Demon was born of us at a certain moment in our lives—divorce, depression, physical and/or sexual abuse, miscarriage, mental and/or verbal abuse, psychological trauma... the list is very long. Far longer than I can hope to address, which has given our enemy a long-held advantage over us... but no more.

The Demon has hidden in Its anonymity too long. You are beginning to see It now, aren't you? The Light is getting a little easier for your eyes to manage. Good... really, you're doing so well. Can you feel it yet? Excellent... let yourself feel it. Things will only get better with your Good Thoughts to protect you. Remember that.

Yet another population of sufferers resides in the caregivers, those who work in the medical fields: nurses, hospice workers, counselors. These are the ones who have Demons whose "Not Good Enough" tirade is reinforced with messages of needing to give more to humanity, to help others, to fix someone else in the vain attempt that someday they too will begin to fill themselves up. You cannot fix enough people in this world to fix yourself. The Demon lies when It promises that. The Demon doesn't really care... not how long a shift you worked without eating, and not the number of patients you were able to treat on any given day with only one meal inside you.

The celebrities who fight this Demon? The rich and the powerful who seem to catch Demons as easily as the rest of us do? Let me give you a glimpse into what their Demons have whispered to them: *You aren't worthy of the success you've got. You have no real talent, and you don't deserve the money, or the fame, or any of it. You're disgusting. All you deserve is to hurt. You're a slut who used her repulsive body to make it to the top. You're a fat, old sow; you're getting so fat and so old, and there's nothing you can do to stop any of it... and that's gonna make you an Untouchable in Hollywood, in Milan..... So throw it up. Try to help. You can try, you worthless pig.*

Glamorous, huh? The glamorous lifestyle of an eating disorder. Really great, I like the part when you get vomit in your hair best. Now that's sexy. Hey laxative abusers? I bet you've got at least one or two "didn't-quite-make-it-in-time" stories you don't want to remember, but do. Talk about attractive! Why the media ever decided this was a glamorous disease is truly beyond me.

(Because they didn't understand the true nature of the Demon is why. They only looked at Its surface and came to their own conclusions in the absence of Light, of Truth).

And, there are yet more behaviors the Demon is teaching us in order to inflict Pain and keep Itself well-fed. The cutters, those who self-inflict wounds, are another dangerous and relatively new cultural phenomenon that the Demons have wreaked upon us. In many ways, I do believe their Demons are no different, only the method of the self-destructive behavior has changed. Sometimes they coalesce, and anorexics are cutters are bulimics. The Pain grows big then. A Demon's feast.

So many of us out there, all in such Pain. So lost in the dark for so long. Fighting desperately, seeking to control our life's experiences and thereby control our destructive and hateful emotions. Hide the Pain. Let no one know. If they do know, pretend It is something you don't care about. Pretend It is no big deal. Pretend It isn't hurting as much as It really is inside.

Stop and breathe. You are not in the darkness any longer, not by a long shot now. Breathing is the key to life; it will build your energy inside. Find time to breathe deeply, from deep in your belly, even if it's just at the red lights in your car.

Breathe. Open your ribcage and ride the breath into your belly. Any time you feel trapped and desperate, you can always begin deep breathing.

Breathing creates energy; it creates the prana that will help you fight the negativity which is combating for your attention inside. Breathe deeply and with awareness. It's free, and it helps more than I can hope to convey. Meditative techniques to spur active intuition and internal visualizations all begin with breathing deeply and with awareness.

Breathe.

Let's review… where did the Demon come from? It came from us, born from a moment of blackest Pain in our lives. Then, It found a way to hang on by getting you to hurt yourself, mentally and physically.

Why does It cause Pain? Because the only way It can grow and maintain Form is to continue to energetically ingest more of the emotion it was born of.

What can you do to rid yourself of it? You make Its atmosphere toxic.

You Love.

A part of you already knows this. I can remember the times when my Demon was in control and people would speak to me in frustration and anger… it was so easy to be angry back. The Demon had me angry all the time, it came natural.

But if someone showed me Love? Took my hand, held me in their arms, and spoke words of Compassion? I melted. I crumbled, my reserves couldn't fight it. I didn't know *how* to fight it. I knew deep inside I didn't even *want* to fight it. But my Demon did.

Picture the child you have been nurturing inside, and give her a hug. Love her; tell her how beautiful and perfect she is, right now. Continue to do this at least once a day, every day. Do it even on the days when you don't think you can say it to yourself and really mean it. Hold her even longer on those days when you *can* find her deep inside. See her face.

The more Love for yourself that you build into your life again, the more you will slowly deprive this Demon of what It's existed off of. And as you do, It *will* begin to collapse. It will begin to control less and less of your thought processes and eventually, your physical actions.

That is to say, if you find yourself reading this and understanding, but so far, you still haven't found a way to stop the behaviors... believe that you can and you will. First you have to shrink your Demon by retraining your emotions. It took time for the Demon to convince you to dig yourself this deeply into the pit, realize it is okay for it to take the time necessary to climb your way back out again. Inch by inch, with intention, just like we said, you will succeed. Be patient and diligent.

Use your imagery of Love, of the child we are protecting, the Authentic Self. Fight the Demon's messages, even as you're bending over and the white of the porcelain is before your eyes. Would you make that loving child do this? Then why... *why* would you continue to do so now? Can you stand up, walk away, take a drive, go shopping, call someone, do anything else but *this*?

Your Demon will shrink if you can learn to disobey Its terrible commands. Begin rebelling now. Be a rebellious fucking bitch to the Demon. Use those claws your Demon gave you and this time, use their deadly sharpness on the Bastard himself. Rebel.

Fight with no one but the Demon. And to fight the Demon most effectively, you must realize Love inside you once more. "Darkness cannot drive out darkness; only light can do that. Hate cannot drive out hate; only love can do that," taught Dr. Martin Luther King, Jr. Now there was a man who understood how to react to Demons... with loving intentions and compassion. The finest Demon weaponry a person can have in their arsenal.

Loving intentions, and compassion. Not for others... for *you*. For the fact that you ate a meal and didn't purge. For the fact that you are never going to be this impossible image of perfection, and only this Demon is trying to make you be. Because once upon a time, long ago, you got hurt... real bad. And from that, the Demon came to be, and the Demon pretended to be You. You thought this desire to hurt yourself came from within yourself. We know now that it didn't. You came from Love.

The more Love you begin to build back into your mind and your emotions, shedding these shackles of lies that the Demon has told you, that only Pain would make you feel better... the easier it becomes to change your mind, and your body, and your behaviors. For good. For real this time.

You shift the energy. My best friend Autumn and I often talk about moving energy in our lives, "Ya gotta shift the energy baby, get rid of all this old stuff and start makin' room for something new."

Something new. Something better. A new way to see yourself, and a new way to see your world. A new way to live. A new way to eat. New choices, in every moment of every day. The choice to notice the promise of a flower and the beauty of a snowflake. To give Love, and to receive Love. To react with Kindness when met with Anger.

Shift the energy. Pull out the negativity and the lower emotions the Demon has made you comfortable with, bit by bit. And then, fill those empty spots with Love. Fight the Pain and Hate with their emotionally polar opposites, with Love and Compassion.

Look up this time when you brush your teeth; look into your eyes again as you do your makeup. Why couldn't you look her in the eyes? The woman there is not hideous, nor shameful. She is the same as we all are, deep down. She's a creature of Light who's reaching towards the Source, to God, to the Divine. She just lost her way for a short while.

Forgive yourself. We are here to make mistakes. As my friend Joanne says, "We're here to break our hearts," because the truth of the Earth realm is that we are here to learn, and perhaps it takes some of us, stubborn as we are, a good long time in the Dark to remember our course back to the Light, the course that always came natural when we were young, before the Pain set in.

Let the Pain be the learning experience, and realize it too is part of your path towards Divinity. You understand now your emotions aren't something to fight, not something you need to control or shut down and ignore; they're just the compass that guides us, giving feedback on how closely aligned we are to Universal Love.

You can begin by observing your emotions in the here and now; as you do, you can learn to retrain them with loving intentions. You have already learned the necessity of realigning them in order to become the person you were meant to be in this life.

It's time to Love yourself again.

The Real You is made of Love.

ஐAnger Management and the Blame Gameஐ

"This is all my fault, it's me she's mad at. She's only doing this to punish us. I don't know why she's so angry all the time. She won't *let* us help her. It's like she blames *us* for everything that's wrong in her life."

Blame and guilt. They are twins, and they have run rampant inside many of us without ever being examined. At times, the tolls that these emotions—Blame, Guilt and Anger—have taken upon our hearts seem insufferable.

Inside, while we have been under the Demon's influence, we have silently grieved to see how our loved ones blame themselves for our problems; we feel incredibly Guilty over the fact that we can't explain ourselves or our actions. We knew we needed to keep everyone away from It, but we understood little else of *why* we're doing what we were doing. So we Blame ourselves even more (creating more Pain) and we feel Guilty about that too.

Yet, behind that Guilt is the rage, the Demon's anger... the Blame we place on others for the Pain we are suffering. We may not know *why* we're blaming others for how we starve and hurt ourselves—we simply seek a target to place the Blame upon, because the Guilt is mounting inside.

And then, there are the times that the Guilt turns inward... when we blame ourselves. For everything. Not just the food, not just the calories. For Everything.

Here is what we might say, our Authentic Selves, if we dare to open our mouths and speak, "I can't live with this Guilt the rest of my life. It's eating me up inside."

And yes, it literally is doing just that. The Guilt makes room for more Pain, and the more Pain you generate, the more your Demon feeds upon it. It is, indeed, eating you up. And starving you to death in the process.

How did it start, how did you *get* your eating disorder, your Demon?

It started with Pain. A thought form is born of the emotion it came from, and can only take in more of what It is. This we know.

The Demon was born of *your* Pain, it is *your* thought form.

For many, the moment of blackest Pain that caused their eating disorder to initially manifest is a time of humiliation, shame, rage and anger. You may have been used, and/or abused, by another (friend, parent, boyfriend, teacher) in any given way… verbally, mentally, emotionally, physically. You may have fallen into a deep depression, by circumstance or by body chemistry, and been unable to shake off the Pain malingering inside.

Pain gave birth to your Demon. And Blame and Guilt are the Demon's tools to manipulate your emotional landscape into one of bleak despair, so that It can live fat and happy in your head. Those emotions do not belong to you; they belong to the Demon.

You've Blamed yourself, and others, and your Guilt has done nothing but cause you and those nearby more Pain. You didn't know the real one to Blame wasn't them, and it wasn't you… it was It.

Why?

The emotions of Blame and Guilt get tangled up inside us as they're encouraged to grow under our Demon's watchful eye. Blame and Guilt cause Pain, and the Demon does love to eat, right?

What the outsiders don't know is how much, deep inside, our Authentic Self silently grieves to see another person walk away, to see that another has given up on us. One more has fallen for the Demon's words and the Demon's tricks; they believed it was the Real You doing and saying those terrible things. They don't know our Authentic Self is locked away inside, and so they fell for the Demon's tricks that we don't know how to stop.

The Demon Forbids us to feel Love. And, we are Forbidden to ask for help.

The Demon cackles when someone gives up on us, especially if It has managed to poison your mind and used your own words to drive them away. Remember how It likes to keep you isolated from others? And, in the absence of help, the Demon twists the knife: *I told you that you were unreachable, unhelpable, and completely* unworthy *of anyone's compassion to begin with. Why should you be so surprised to see another person leave you? You're disgusting. The only one who isn't leaving you is* ME.

Blame and Guilt. We're gonna flex your emotional intelligence muscles some more in this chapter. The Light is really getting nice now, isn't it? A soft warm glow, one that can penetrate the years of cold emotional barriers you've put around your poor, broken heart. Let's think about the Pain, and see if you can find your way through this tangle inside.

As a student of Tantra, I've learned to question the purpose of an emotion as it presents itself inside me, "What are you here to teach me about myself?" Tantra teaches us that our emotions are tools, built-in instructions on how we can advance our soul along our path. As we've established, they provide constant feedback for our soul's journey… where are we today, what is our proximity to the Source? What level are we operating on; is it one of the higher emotions, or are we still operating from deep inside the pits of despair?

How do we feel today? And how do those emotions propel our soul's path forward to the Light?

Logically, positive emotions are easy for us to recognize as helping us. But, what about negative ones I asked of my Angels, my Teachers, in meditation. Aren't they detrimental? Isn't a path towards the Source one which encompasses only the higher vibratory emotions anyhow? So if that's the case, I argued internally, why do we experience any lower emotions, ever? They're only dragging us back down. Hindering our path. Right?

Their answer? *Every* emotion comes from a sacred Source within us, and that Source is our soul, our connection to God. The emotions, all of them, good and bad, are meant to instruct us on our path. Emotions are messages from our soul, and as such are not meant to be ignored.

This is why you cannot just *ignore* your problem; it's why you want help out of the hell you're in. Behind the emotions of habitual acceptance to the Demon's Rules, there is the soul's cry for help and the anguishing feeling of sinking below the waters for the final time.

"Alright, emotions come from my soul. But what's this 'Teachers' stuff, Alissa?"

When I pray, I begin to breathe deeply and quiet my mind to listen inwardly for spiritual guidance. It is my firm belief that all of us, every single one, have Teachers who are with us all our lives—we may call them Guardian Angels, or in some religions, we may believe our Ancestors' spirits are guiding us with their wisdom. Regardless, I believe in spiritual helpers, interceders between me, down here in the material realm, and the ultimate Source, which I travel towards, along with everything and everybody else in the Universe. Our Teachers' purpose is to assist our path towards the Light should we chose to call upon them for guidance in moments of meditation and prayer.

"Well, everyone's got 'em but *me*. I've never heard a single thing from *any* of my supposed Teachers, Alissa. So, are they on permanent vacation or what, because I could use some help right about now!"

A dialogue with your Teachers, your Angels, is up to *you* to begin. To my understanding, your Teachers are like reference sources. Unless you go and look up what you need in a dictionary, it won't actively offer you any information—Inner Teachers work the same. You gotta pick up the phone first. Your Teachers are your references; they are here to help you and can be communicated with through your focused thoughts, meditations and prayers. But, they do not *initiate* the interior dialogue. We do.

To practice this, find times when you can quiet yourself and focus inwardly. Breathe deeply, expanding from the belly and not the chest, and let your mind let go of its jumpy-monkey thoughts ("I have a paper due on Thursday. If I don't pick up the dry cleaning tonight, I'll have to swing by tomorrow.") Breathe until you calm down, focus on the feeling of your breath moving in and out as a replacement for all of your other thoughts. Listen to the sounds around you, how many can you hear when you grow quiet enough? How many are in the room you sit in? How many outside? Active listening will quiet the jumpy-monkey mind nicely when given some breathing and time.

Once you have centered yourself and your mind is quiet, you can begin the discussion. How? You pray. You meditate. You open your mind and try to let go of analytical thought. Let images come to you; do not question things that begin to flit by in your mind. If you have something specific, focus your thoughts on the issue and ask for your Teachers' assistance. The interior voice that Angels use is sometimes hard to hear until we're really quiet inside. Seek and you will find; knock and the door will be opened.

Breathe.

So, let's examine the first emotion here… what is Blame? Blaming is the emotional attempt to persuade another to feel Guilt; it is emotional coercion for the purpose of giving us a sense of power. Blaming is most often an "active" emotion in that it seeks *outwardly* for a source to provide its false feeling of emotional control—we convince another of their Guilt by blaming them for something… that is to say, by hurting another, we feel stronger.

"You broke my best dish! My grandmother gave that to me, and she's dead. You ruined it!" A statement such as this uses Blame to place the emotion of Guilt, and therefore Pain, inside someone else. The goal of this action is to spread some of the Pain we are experiencing—we can spread it, but doing so does not shed it. Blaming is a futile attempt to gain back power.

Blame is like taking a kid's candy away… except instead of candy, we're taking away their good feelings, and trying to replace them with what we think they should be feeling… that is, Guilt.

Have you looked at yourself and blamed your problems on others? "It's all my mother's/father's/abuser's/boyfriend's/husband's/brother's/sister's fault… if they hadn't done this to me, I wouldn't be so screwed up now!"

Why were you blaming them? Because you tried to take your Pain and give part of it to someone else. You probably thought (without actively examining such thoughts) that pushing part of the hurt onto another would bring you some sort of screwed up relief. And with the Demon calling the shots, of course it didn't. Momentary grim and hateful satisfaction, maybe. Those are acceptable by the Demon's terms, but real relief? Oh no….

By blaming others, you are trying to insert your Pain into another person as an attempt to alleviate what you're feeling. That doesn't work, and you know it. If it did, we would have cured ourselves of our Demon long ago. But, it does make us feel temporarily powerful to hurt another, especially if we have been hurting for so long. And, in doing so, we create more internal Pain for the Demon.

And then there are those whom the Demon likes to persuade to blame themselves. "I'm the only person in this world as exquisitely screwed up as I am, I deserve all this." Here is an even more futile attempt at relief—instead of seeking another person to give part of our hurt to, we place the hurt (Blame) back on ourselves. Why? The Demon just created a nice black pit of emotions there to suck on too, eh? Active or passive, Blame spreads Pain.

Let us use another hypothetical example: "If he hadn't raped me, I wouldn't be killing myself by starving every day. I hate myself, and it's his fault for making me hate ME so damn much."

This is Blame. This is the attempt to justify the hurt we've dealt with, and to insert some of that hurt back into another—in this case, back into the perpetrator of the Pain.

Now just stop and think on this alone… is it really so *wrong* to blame a person who has legitimately hurt you? No, it's *not*. It's good. It works to your ultimate benefit. That is why Blame is an essential emotion to your soul's path. Blame is the ability to recognize the source of your pain, and letting that source know that you feel they are responsible.

Intention is everything, examine the person you are blaming and their intentions at the time they acted against you—a rapist *meant* to cause this pain, it was their Intention by doing this act. Therefore, they *deserve* the Blame we are feeling.

Blame itself is not always bad. It is how Blame interacts with our path to the Source, to Love, that can make it good or bad.

Blame can *help* us along on our soul's path. Every emotion, regardless of what vibration it travels at (be it high or low) is meant to help you. And the ability to recognize those who have caused you pain so you can avoid more of the same is how Blame can *help* you, and why Blame is a necessary part of the human experience.

Blame can help you identify the Source of your Pain, but only if you're very honest with yourself.

Blame is really easy to go overboard on. "My parents screwed me up with all their expectations, and my teachers are always pushing me to do more, and my friends don't understand me, and my boyfriend only uses me for sex...."

Are all these people *really* the source of your pain? Or, in this case, has the emotion of Blame let you feel important by spreading it around to everyone you can?

Blame which imparts a sense of Guilt into another as a means of hurting or feeling powerful causes Pain; it hurts others, which makes Blame bad. Blame can help us to recognize those who have done us harm so that we may better avoid them; it helps us heal, which makes Blame good.

Blame is necessary, and Guilt is necessary to the human experience in order to propel our soul's path to the Light. They are not emotions for you to stuff away, to ignore and pretend they'll go away. You feel Guilt every time you swallow food... and you think you can forget about it? The Demon won't allow that, not while It gets to call the shots.

Okay, Teachers, I said... that's why we Blame others, and maybe even why the Demon gets us to Blame ourselves... to give It more emotional power. That much I supposed I could accept. But, that was only the tip of the iceberg.

Blaming is very active, like anger is active. In acting, I learned to hone my Tantric ability of "emotional excavation". I would be given a script, and then—like any actor—I would try to uncover *why* did my character feel the way she did, and therefore *why* did she say these things, and take these actions in her life? This is the process that actors call "discovering their character's 'motivation.'"

Motivation and Intention are very closely linked, remember that.

But for now, dissecting a script for character analyzation is not unlike learning to dissect yourself. *Why did I just say that? Why am I feeling so (angry, upset, scared, happy) right now? What just happened to get me to feel so strongly, and why? What did it trigger inside me? What event did it remind me of, what associations did I jump to, however fleetingly?*

By the way, look up real quick... see that Light in the distance that's calling you? Guess what? It's not a train. You keep thinking about that Light, and I'll just keep talking.

Back to the Teachers' lessons. One thing my Inner Teachers taught me, during script-inspired emotional digging, was an emotional truth that rocked me to the core.

Anger always masks Fear.

Why does a character get angry? Because they're *afraid* of something.

An actor can *not* go out onstage and be AngryMan, or AngryWoman, and expect that to be believable to an audience. Why is that? Because anger for anger's sake is flat, that's why. Anger is something else.... Anger is the emotion that lets us feel In Control when we sense danger. Anger is an emotional self-defense mechanism.

Example: A car swerves in front of me on the freeway and I slam on my brakes, narrowly avoiding an accident. As a result, I scream and rage, and feel blind fury for this other person.

I was scared to death, and felt out of control. And so, I got mad.

Anger Always Masks Fear. Anger is an active emotion, it broils and gets us very wrapped up in it; we say we are consumed with our anger. We let it come flooding into us, without reserve. But why?

Anger gives us our sense of power back, just as Blame gives us our sense of power back. Anger is taking control of the situation, and fear is when we are definitely *not* in control. Anger steps in to help us, in some measure, to take action.

And action is often what will literally save our lives. The action you took to read this book, for example.

Anger *is* a very useful emotion indeed. All emotions are useful, all come from the Source for a reason. Even if it takes some digging to find those reasons. Anger acts as the catalyst to action. Action can save our lives. This is why I teach you now to use the anger you are so used to feeling, but to turn it on the Demon instead of on yourself. Anger helps. Anger is a self defense mechanism that each of us carries, and it's literally as deeply ingrained as fight or flight. Fight or flight, anger or panic, is the basic instinct that will often save your ass.

Flight... panic is the emotional opposite of Anger. Panic is Fear. Panic is the ultimate realization that you are horribly *out of control* of a very dangerous situation. Anger is the attempt to *take control* of a very dangerous situation.

Anger always masks Fear, and Panic is Fear's unmasking. And both emotions serve a purpose which is meant to assist our ultimate path, or we wouldn't experience them.

So... if this is true... why Guilt? What purpose does Guilt serve?

Guilt, guilt, guilt. The emotion that everyone says, "Oh what a waste of time it is to feel guilty. Just flush that Guilt, get rid of it, it's a waste of your energy." As tempting as that may be, it is also not the correct way to handle Guilt. That is tantamount to saying, "I don't care how I really feel, I just don't want to feel uncomfortable—and this Guilt is uncomfortable, so I don't like it and I'm getting rid of it."

To deny or suppress our emotions is not the same as learning from them. It does not release them. Only when we embrace our emotions can we experience the lessons they inherently are, and allow them to propel us closer to the Source. As long as we deny, suppress, medicate, and in any other way try to ignore how we are feeling, we are not listening to the messages from our soul.

But, dammit Teachers... that means we humans have to experience all of our emotions, not just the good ones! The really crappyass ones too. So, WHY??? Our path is to the Source, groovy Love and Bliss, ain't it? Why should we hurt? Ever?

On one very frustrating day, I absolutely *demanded* to be told why Guilt was a human emotion—what could possibly be the purpose of such a horrible, hurtful state of mind? What does this emotion teach us, what purpose does it serve humanity besides hurting us?

Guilt is a pointer, the same as Anger, my Teachers answered. Anger points to what we Fear. Guilt is here to teach you about what you Love.

No, that can't be right. What? (You see, I argue with my Teachers as much as you may be arguing with me as you read this. It's the Socratic method, questions are good).

Guilt teaches us what we Love. Doesn't seem right, on the surface, does it?

Guilt feels terrible, Love feels great. How can they be related? Remember when I told you a while back that Intention is everything? Here's where we're gonna really start to explore that.

Guilt points its finger not at us, but at what we cherish. If we have not taken a moment to realize the importance of that thing, Guilt reminds us to. Hard to follow? Here's an example: a girl cheats on her boyfriend. Afterwards, she feels guilty.

The Guilt she feels is pointing her attention to that which she Loves.

The ultimate purpose of Guilt, said my Teachers, is to teach us Compassion. As a species, to advance us towards the Light.

The Guilt pointed her attention to what she values. Her Guilt is reminding her of what is really important. Ultimately, Guilt points us to discover what it is we truly care for… what we Love. By realizing her culpability, Guilt builds her compassion as she recognizes the Pain her actions have caused.

Guilt is ultimately meant to propel us closer to Love, to the Source.

In this example, it could be she truly loves her boyfriend and feels Guilt reminding her of that, so that she will learn to cherish what she Loves. Maybe she doesn't love her boyfriend, but she does feel she let herself down as a person… morally. And that perception of her own failure inspires her Guilt—she lost her sense of feeling morally good, her connection to the Source.

Either way, Guilt is pointing to what she cherishes, to something of personal value. Guilt should never simply be disregarded and treated like flotsam to dispose of; the key to managing Guilt is to take a moment to follow the pointer.

"I feel Guilty because I ditched class today," says the college student. Why? The Guilt is pointing to the fact that you truly value learning, that you want to achieve good grades to feel good about yourself, or perhaps you value your college money and know you wasted it by ditching class. Again, the emotion points to that which you value, to that which you Love.

Learn to recognize what Guilt wants to teach you, and you can manage its place in your life and thereby release it. If the Guilt you feel is *not* teaching you things, then it is perhaps time to realize this emotion is not serving a useful purpose. This too will release it.

"But didn't you just say Guilt always serves a purpose?"

Let us review… when we are thinking, we are creating a thought form that coexists with us, with all that we are. A thought form cannot advance Itself beyond what It was at the time of Its creation as set by us, the Creator.

A thought born of Love knows only Love and needs Love to grow bigger. A thought form born of Pain exists on our Pain, and gets very sneaky and manipulative to perpetuate what It needs.

Because Guilt is born of the lower emotions, it can get very tangled up. It can inspire anger, and it can inspire remorse. These too are lower emotions, and we know the more you feed negativity with additional negativity, the larger it grows.

When Guilt inspires anything but Compassion and Love, it is no longer useful. It should be recognized as such, and thereby released.

"I feel terrible. I should have returned this casserole dish last week." What is the Guilt teaching us? I value my friend's opinion of me, and I fear it was negatively impacted by these actions I've done. Can you remedy this?

Of course you can.

"I feel really guilty—I put butter on the baked potato I ate over lunch." What is the Guilt teaching you here? What Love does it point to? That we love to listen to the Demon's Rules? That butter is the enemy? Or is this an example of wasteful Guilt? What was your Intention when you ate that baked potato, to feed your body and enjoy the nourishment in a way that was delicious… or will you let the Demon place Its Blame and Guilt into your heart, needlessly, so It can produce more Pain inside you?

Follow it out… follow it out. Tantra is the gift of our emotional selves. Honor the gifts your emotions hold, and learn to recognize their lessons. This can help you put Guilt in its proper and honorable place in your life.

Intention is everything. Our intentions create the thought forms that surround us. We dictate what we will attract and repel, and continue to harmonize this by our ongoing emotions and thoughts, as well as the physical, real-world experiences we have on any given day. We may not be able to change the past, and all the actions that were already taken. But we can change how we feel about it, today.

Once, I saw on TV a psychologist interviewing a mother whose son had died. The mother had left her adolescent son in the car while running inside to quickly finish an errand, and in her absence, the boy had played with the gear shift. When the car began to roll, he panicked, and jumped out to try and stop the car. When he was killed in the process, her Guilt knew no end.

Every day, there was her Guilt. There was all that she had done wrong, every bad decision and all that it had cost her, and would continue to cost her, every day that she lived and her son did not.

What was the Guilt teaching her, what did it point to? Her Love for her son. At the most terrible emotional cost any parent could ever bare to imagine.

Guilt wasn't part of her life to ruin her, to punish her. And yet, its daily presence was causing her to withdraw from her husband and other children, shielding herself from the Pain she believed she would cause others. The Guilt was tangled deeply inside her grief, and once buried there, It did not seek to be released.

Like an eating disorder, her Guilt, her Demon, was given a place to grow. And It lived off her Pain, and the Pain It continued to inflict upon her, daily, until the moment when It would finally suck her dry.

But, the psychologist knew how to help her, and encouraged the mother to reflect on her Intention at the moment of the accident.

Intention is everything. When we set our Intention, we can use this as a gauge for the usefulness of our Guilt. Was it this mother's Intention to cause her son this grievous death?

No. Her Intention was to run the errand quickly and return. She believed her son would be fine, that he was old enough to know better than to take the actions he did. She did not Intend to cause this accident. It simply happened. Her Guilt had taught her all it could about what she Loved.

And so, she could begin to release It. It does no good to Blame the victim. Inserting Guilt into the victim no longer assists in propelling us towards the Source. Example: an abused child blames herself for her molester's deeds. Was it her Intention to reap such grievous results in her life at that time? Or was she simply Guilty of the sin of being vulnerable?

And what does her Guilt teach her? How much she valued and loved her innocent self.

The Blame, and the Guilt... all that you have carried inside you, all that you have done to others.... Now is the time to examine these emotions, and their true causes, with the Light I've shared.

The Flashlight is really getting bright now. I'm glad... you look so beautiful in the Light.

Blame is the process of trying to make ourselves feel powerful by inserting Guilt into another.

Anger is a mask, and it hides the fear we are feeling, in order to gain control of what feels dangerously out of control.

Panic is the recognition of a dangerous situation and the realization of our inability to prevent anticipated Pain.

And Guilt teaches us Compassion for what we Love.

You've just had Emotional Excavation Training 101, now it's time for you to dig inside yourself. Sift through the fertile topsoil of your mind until you find the place inside where the quiet answers lie and the heartache melts away. Dig through the layers of Pain, and examine your intentions for all that still hurts you inside. Was it really your fault? Can you quit blaming yourself for it now?

Your emotions can be used to your advantage, just as they were always meant to be. You set your Intentions, every moment of every day, with every thought, however big or small. Let your Intentions be those of the higher emotions, and you will begin to feel more Love in your life again.

Love is the only thing can drive away the Demon, to starve It of Its banquet of Pain and to deny It the atmosphere of Hate which It needs to live.

Before we go... I've got one more thing to talk to you about. That "Control" issue you've had. Actually, the Control issue you *thought* you needed to have, because your Demon told you so.

"I can't control my life; I can't control how I feel, and all I feel is Pain! I can't stop crying! I need some self-control!"

Your Demon rubbed your nose in the Pain It was born from, and grew inside of you a toxic dump of emotions for It to live off of. And did the Demon even say thank you for the emotional hell you're supporting It with? Oh nooooo… the Demon said, "Look at what *you* did, you're out of control!"

And here, little fatty, is how you can be back *in* control… here's your Hoop. Start jumping.

Starve, starve, binge, purge, cry, purge, starve, weep. That wasn't control. You thought it was because the Demon taught you restriction and Pain equaled self-control. Why? Because It wanted you to hurt. So It could grow.

How many times have I heard the psychological theory, "an eating disorder is a patient's attempt to gain a sense of control over their lives, and in doing so, improve their self-image." What the hell? *I* didn't do this at all… the Demon did this to me! It was the Demon who taught me to live in a perpetual state of Anger and Panic, Guilt and Rage.

The Demon has us scared to death! Panic set in and to deal with that we repeat the mantra, "Control… control." Instead of judging for ourselves, we gave our power to the scale and let it tell us if we're doing a good job controlling our lives or not.

Why?

Your Demon let you feel Panic for the emotions you carried every day in order for It to survive. Instead of thanking you for your Pain, your Demon said, "You need to control your life, and you can start by doing this…." And so, it all began.

Control is not Panic. As we just discussed, Panic is the recognition of a dangerous situation and realizing our inability to prevent anticipated Pain. The Demon wants you to Panic to make you anticipate Pain, which It needs and loves. Therefore, Panic is what you feel when you step on the scale after a big meal you allowed yourself to eat. It's Panic to swallow bites of food.

The sense of being "out of control" comes from the Demon. As long as you believe you are out of control of your life, you are susceptible to allowing someone or some Thing else control you instead. Which is why the Demon preaches "no control, no control!" at you all day long. To do so subtly reinforces Its position of power; it strengthens the false sense of command that the coping mechanisms of hurting and starving present us.

The scale becomes the only metaphor which gauges your self-control. The Demon told you that you had to learn to control yourself. The Demon then created an atmosphere of emotional hell so you would be sure to fail, and in doing so, would feel even worse. The scale became your compass instead of your emotions. That way, the Demon was sure to drag you down, down, down… thinner, thinner, more Pain, more….

Your emotions don't need controlled, and you don't need to "get a handle on your emotions." Your emotions need to be embraced, and I've explained why—not just the positive ones, but even the negative emotions. This whole chapter has already taught you why your emotions are essential to your soul's path, which is why we left this "Control" thing to look at last. You needed time for your eyes to adjust to the Light, just as they have.

And you are so incredibly beautiful, do not be afraid. Your heart is safe and will remain so until the day you can unlock the Demon's cage and put that stinking bastard inside instead. You don't need to control your emotions. You don't need to control your food choices. You don't need to control your weight as some futile, fucked up way of controlling the Demon.

The only thing in your life that needed controlled was the horrifying reign of the Demon, but It cast Its spell on you so you'd never see that. You'd just punish yourself, and others, instead of realizing It was the monster that started it all.

It's the Demon that needs locked in the box. Your heart needs out.

You *are* In Control.

❧Caging the Demon by Breaking Its Rules☙

This chapter could also be called, "Removing the Hoops." We know our Demon's Rules intimately; for years, we've added to them in variations and minuets that would make even the great composers weep. But we also have practiced examining those Rules, first by writing them out. Writing the Rules allowed us to see how pitiful, illogical and ridiculous they really are when we take them out of our head and put them somewhere else instead.

Then, we learned to speak our defense arguments to the Demon. Instead of continuing the fight with ourselves, we began to fight back against It instead, and in doing so, you have already started the process of Breaking the Rules. We've *already* proven the fact that the Rules can be broken... but it's a scary process when old paradigms come crumbling down.

Ultimately, you *know* you need to destroy the house that the Demon has made inside in order to truly be free of Its insidious grasp. But... it's freaking scary, isn't it? I'm talking Terrifying to even consider kinda scary. Believe it or not, that's *good*. It means you're on the right track.

In the Tarot deck, there is a card called "The Tower." In older decks, it was also called "Le Maison Dieu," the House of God. A lightning bolt is commonly seen striking at the top of a large building, bricks are falling from the sky—a whole way of life is violently exploding, and the people in the card are free-falling in midair, propelled unforgivingly from their confining yet comfortable place inside the Tower by this Source of Divine Light.

Your own Tower must come tumbling down. Light *is* Truth, and the Tower's lightning bolt is Zeus hurling the Truth right smack into your world. Light illuminates, it shows us the Truth; without Light, we cannot see things for how they really are. I am giving you a new Light, a new Truth, to examine your eating disorder with; as a result, now you can see It in a totally new way. Nothing evil can ever withstand the power of Divine Light. Divinity, Light and Truth are synonymous. And the Tower represents the Demon's prison of darkness and lies that you've been kept prisoner inside.

The Tower card is often compared to the Tower of Babel in the Bible, when the word of God touched upon the people and suddenly they could all understand the many languages spoken around them. The Truth was revealed to all in a blinding moment of Illumination that destroyed all of their previously held notions. Truth irrevocably changed their world view forever. Nothing would ever be the same. The bricks came tumbling down.

If you look at the divinatory interpretations for the card, you will learn the Tower foretells of a time of destruction, that old paradigms and belief systems are crashing, big time. When the Tower appears, your entire world is literally falling apart; the destruction feels like an act of God that you couldn't possibly control, and now you're free-falling to what seems to be your imminent death. You're certain this is the end.

But it's not. The Tower *is* destruction, but it is *not* the end.

I noticed something about the Tower in my Tarot studies. If you examine the Ace of Cups card from the Waite-Colman-Smith Tarot deck, you may notice how much the base of that cup looks like the Tower before it was struck by lightning. Now flip back to card 16 and check out the base of the Tower. Why, the base is the only part of the whole structure that *doesn't* come crumbling down!

What does this teach us? That which is built on the energy of the Ace of Cups card—Love, Compassion, and the seed of Hope—can withstand the destructive forces that assail.

Illumination doesn't strike upon us to hurt us; it comes when we are ready to shake our world apart and start again. To build on what remains… on Truth, and on that which we made with the bricks of Compassion and Love in our lives.

We rebuild our lives with authenticity. With integrity.

Breaking the habits of your day, the starving or purging cycles that you are so comfortable living with, is like living through the Tower card. You are destroying that which you know, that which has stood for a long time as *who you are*. The Hoops of your day—the number of times you check the scale, the number of minutes you work out, the number of calories you're "allowed" to eat—all of these are *your* behaviors to discard. No one but you can *make* you stop. Others can send you to counselors, or hook you up to IVs and force feed you back into your body, but no one else can *really* make you stop doing what the Demon's been demanding... except you.

So, why does it feel so difficult to do? If we can accept that the Demon's reign is over, and we realize that *we* are ultimately in control of our body, and we even realize that the Demon's lies aren't to be accepted as a way of life... why is it still so hard to take over again?

Because the physical acts that were repeated over time have been made into an identity. And by changing those acts, you begin to change your identity.

And your Demon doesn't want you to change.

The part of you that's fighting even still, the part that's scared to death to make the change, the part that's screaming in fear, "I'll get fat! I'll get fat!", that part doesn't know how to run your life very well... but even so, it doesn't want to let go of its control of you either, does it?

Too bad. It's time for it to go. The walls are gonna come tumbling down.

"Alissa, there's a terrible comfort in just deciding to remain this screwed up, you know? I mean, I hate this eating disorder, this Demon as you say. But... I dunno if I can really... just stop...."

You *can*. You've already started. You created a new vision of yourself several chapters ago when you began to see yourself, your Authentic Self, as a precious child under your care. You opened yourself to this new thought form, and every time you've gone back to her in your mind as the Demon's voice rails in your head, you've given strength to that new thought form, to that precious baby girl, the Real You.

Your metamorphosis has already begun. It's scary. It's like walking over that cliff edge the first time you go repelling, it's *scary* and every instinct inside is waving red flags, "Wrong! Wrong! No can do! STOP!"

Why is it this scary? Why does it seem to cause us such full-scale Panic to think about getting healthy, about eating?

Because the Demon is Panicking… big time. It's the Demon's Fear we feel, and as the paradigm that's kept the Bastard in control begins to crumble and give way, you better believe It's going to fight and fight and use every emotional hold over you that It still has to try to get you to STOP GETTING BETTER!

You get better… It dies. It doesn't want that. It knows how to manipulate your thoughts and emotions, and will try to freak you back into your diseased-thinking. The more you continue taking control again, the more It freaks and freaks and pushes Panic buttons in your head. Panic buttons *you* didn't even knew you had. Why? It doesn't *want* you in control; It knows that you might get rid of It if you were calling the shots in your life instead.

In order for you to get better, one identity *will* die. It's not just the internal voice of the Demon that has to go. It's the old You too. You have to flush all of the dysfunctional behaviors that you have learned to identify as being who you are.

It's *not* who you are. You're the Real You. You're *not* the Demon. The Demon created this dysfunctional version of the Real You. For your Authentic Self to take control of the physical realm once more there's got to be no one else at the command station.

The You that's very accustomed to living under these inane Rules every single day of her life? Say buh-bye.

You will lose one person, one identity, in the process of recovering—the one that's been controlled by the Demon. This is who we see free-falling in the Tower card, she was propelled to her doom—the old you, the Demonized you. I can guarantee you there will be more than a few days where you will feel upside and sideways… free-falling as the Rules go but stay but go but stay but go.

And yet the Authentic Self, the identity that was built upon Love and Compassion remains safe. It has been tested greatly, and yet she withstands, and waits for you to set her free… for you to destroy the Tower she's been locked inside.

I love that line in *Batman Begins*, "Why do we fall down? So we can learn to pick ourselves back up again." So you fell down. So you let this Demon's tricks take over for a while in your life, maybe even a long while. Instead of beating the crap outta yourself with the usual "I'm worthless, fat and ugly" tirade, why not turn that anger and dissatisfaction against the Demon, just as I've taught you to?

"Destruction sounds… well, destructive! I don't know if I can deal with that kinda of restructuring of my life, I just don't know if I can handle it. It sounds really painful, and I'm in so much pain already. I can't take any more!"

Consider this… what is the purpose of the Tower card, is it meant only to cause us Pain? What does it teach us about the human condition?

The Tower card appears when we are ready for the Light, ready for Divine illumination and understanding to break apart the Tower of darkness, confusion and despair. When we're ready to do away with the isolation and chaos of the Demon, the Tower card appears to set us free from the lies we've accepted for too long. It also says to us, "And now there's no going back."

Here's another archetypal Tower image for you to consider. Victorians made a symbol of King Arthur's "Lady of Shallott," a maiden who was imprisoned within a tower, unable to interact with the real world, unable to do anything but observe it through a *looking glass* from within her ivory cage. She longs with all her heart to be free, yet she knows her imprisonment is her choice, that at any time she could leave. And yet, as soon as she leaves, she will die… she knows this too.

By the poem's end, her choice to leave the Tower, and her death afterwards, allowed her to reclaim her abilities, and to move her soul towards Love. One identity died.

The fear you feel is the subconscious realization that you are very literally killing off a part of yourself. For you to get better, for you to kick this Demon's ass back to hell where It belongs, an identity (for good or bad) which has "helped" you to get by is going away, for good. And it's *hard*. If giving up our crutches and vices were easy, there wouldn't be so many 12-step programs, would there?

The Tarot's Tower card becomes a symbol for your body, and the lightning bolt the symbol for Truth, for the Source; Truth is the ultimate Source of illumination behind this Flashlight I've given you.

This book has been your Flashlight, and allows the Light within to show you what is real, and what are the Demon's illusions.

You have a whole new way of looking at the "eating disorder" now than you did when you began reading. With this new understanding of the Demon, you have already begun to shift your paradigm, and in the process, it feels like you're free-falling in midair to your doom. The Demon is playing on your fears, and seeking to stay in Control and create more Pain for you to live through.

Which is to say, you're scaring the shit outta It right now; how cool is *that?*

Your body and your mind have been divided, like the people of Babel. You are reuniting them, and you've been told by your Demon that such an act is utterly impossible. So impossible, It doesn't even want you *think* about getting better.

But you're thinking about it… right now. You and I, we're creating that thought form inside you too—the vision of "getting healthy." And the more energy you give to the thoughts of recovery, the more energy you steal from the thoughts of despair. (And so the Demon shrinks).

I told you from the beginning, you *will* know fear as you learn to heal yourself. The fear becomes intense as you begin to Remove the Hoops, and Break the Rules. Why? The fear comes from the Demon. It's launching every grenade It still has in Its arsenal to get this healing process to simply *end*.

Always trying to convince you that It and You are One and the Same, the Demon turns Its fear into something that is "yours"–the fear that you are losing control of your body, that you're gonna get fat, that others will stop loving you, that you don't know who to be, or what to do. How will you spend your time if you don't have your purging to structure your entire day around?

Build with Love and Compassion. (Remember that child we've been taking care of, protecting her from the messages of the Demon?) See the child's face within you, and protect her... build her a world of Love and Compassion, for the day she's ready to step forth and take over once more. You've already been holding her and telling her that you Love her. Now it's time to create a world where she can come out and play again.

How?

Break the Demon's Rules. Take back your power, no matter how frightening it seems. Which Hoop are you ready to set down today? Right now? Can you learn to turn the Hate inside you against the Demon and Its demands, instead of upon yourself as you have for so long? Can you turn your anger into something holy and righteous, a jihad for your own Authentic Self? What if instead of pretending to be "ana's lover" all the time you became "ana's worst fucking nightmare" instead?

Here's one Hoop to consider for discarding... Rule Number One.

One very important Rule you need to break, if you haven't already, is the code of Silence that you've been under—it's the Rosicrucian saying again, "Thoughts are things and words have wings." It is time to allow the words from inside you into the open air; it is time to let go of your terrible need to hold this secret inside, open the cage and let your words fly free.

Words have wings. They fly and lift you into flight as well. Are you ready? Of course you're scared; I didn't ask you if you were *scared*. I asked you, are you ready? Because no one else in the world can answer that except *You*.

"So what, everyone knows I have an eating disorder already. It's not a big secret in *my* life, Alissa."

I know what secret *is* a big deal... I know what you never told those others, the ones who know you have an "eating disorder". You never dared to admit the amount of Pain the Demon has sowed in your soul. You've never admitted to *anyone* the Hurt you've lived through, the hell that is the Demon's voice, every minute of every day. The Demon made you hide that, no matter *what* other people think they know of you and your struggle.

...You have tears in your eyes, my beautiful girl. It's okay to cry, tears will melt the bars that have held you in this prison; tears of acceptance will heal. Tears of self-rage and shame are what the Demon taught you to cry. These tears are different; tears of acceptance will raise your vibratory level towards the higher emotions, dissolving the Demon's monument of pain inside. Cry as much as you need to, and then cry a little more.

I will not leave you, I will not go. I'm right here. And unlike so many others, I really do *know* how much it hurts. That's why I wrote this book, after all. Because I knew firsthand and even if I myself had recovered, I couldn't live my life knowing so many of my sisters and brothers were still drowning in the Pain.

Your Demon has taught you that you must suffer alone, in silence, that you are not worthy of help. The Demon cannot bear Love. Like we said, hatred and anger the Voice can deal with all day, any day. But when someone shows you kindness... you melt, right? It's hard to receive kindness, it almost hurts. Your Demon has taught you to hate kindness, but you know inside that isn't really right.

You're free-falling. None of the Rules make sense, none of the Demon's promises are ever kept, nothing makes you feel good about yourself, and no one knows how alone you've been during this struggle.

So, let them in. Break the Demon's Rules.

Breaking the Rules, definitely breaking the code of Demon-imposed silence, is heart wrenching and so *so* scary! It's almost like you expect a safe to fall on your head outta nowhere... random punishment! But remember what I taught you about the Devil card in Tarot, the Great

Liar. The Demon is not *You*, and *It is Lying To You* to keep you *alone* and *helpless* in Its shackles, forever.

These behaviors aren't yours either, they aren't from you. You *can* exist without them, even though the Demon has had a long time to insist otherwise. The word "fat" is how It controls you. In the Devil card, it is up to *us* to realize we put these chains on, and only we can take them back off again. The Demon showed us our Hoops, but only you can decide when it's time to stop jumping through them.

Be forewarned, the Demon can change shapes; It is a master shapeshifter. Often, when one destructive behavior is given up, another replaces it, or several, that are just as destructive if not more so. The Authentic Self will need you to remain vigilant while your Soul slowly continues to take over the vehicle of your body and mind once again.

Watch the Demon, stop it from metamorphing into other Demons, such as alcoholism, drug addiction or sexual abuse (be that promiscuous sex that abuses the Self, or by abusing others). Picking fights to provoke loved ones, throwing blows just so someone can punish you from the outside. Suicidal attempts. Any self destructive behavior that replaces another is not true growth. It isn't a true step towards health, towards the Divine Light that we instinctually crave.

You have learned the first lesson already… that the Voice *can* be denied. That the Voice is Not You. That there is a way back. And the road itself will be walked by no one *but* you. I can show you all the landmarks and give you this neat Flashlight to help you see your way… but I can't move your feet. Only you can.

"Alissa, I'm one of the ones who can't admit to *anyone* that this is really happening. It took me this long just to admit it to MYSELF! There's no way I can tell someone else, they'll hate me!"

Demon talk. Anyone in your life who hates you for saying, "I need to talk," isn't worth having in your life anyhow. So stop the excuses, okay? Alissa's heard 'em, cuz Alissa's Demon spun them once upon a time too.

It's time to take action. You've been fighting for your Authentic Self, and you're getting so much stronger now, can you feel it? The Light in your eyes is coming back, and it isn't the perverted glimmer of the Demon's any more inside that I see. It is so beautiful… your Light inside, how could the Demon have done this to you, my sweet one?

Let's recap some more, you need to stop and look backwards a lot to see you're moving forward. You've *already* learned how to fight the Demon on the energetic level–by starving It of Hate and connecting to your higher emotions instead. But, that's how you fight the Demon on the emotional realm. How do you fight your Demon in the real world?

When you've written everything out, the Rules, the Name-calling, all of it, you've started the real world battle already too. Continue that by *telling someone*. Take the action to break the silence… for real this time. Not just in hidden blogs and journals, not in all the places that are dark enough to hide how much *bad* you've done to yourself.

Find the person in your life that can listen the best, and go have some coffee together. Or, call them. Or, drop by her apartment for no reason. Today. Right now. I don't mind waiting, really–go for it; do it before you chicken out. Get your bookmark; I'll be here when you get back.

"But, Alissa, I don't know what to say! How do I even begin a conversation like that? 'Nice weather we're having, oh by the way. Did you know I make myself throw up four times a day 'cuz I have what Alissa calls a "Demon" inside me?' Nice… they'll run for the hills!"

That's the Demon pushing another Panic button. Telling you that you *can't*. Like always. Using (and manipulating) your emotions in order to reinforce Rule Number One: You Cannot Say Anything.

Do you see now? Do you see how easy it is to pick out the Demon's lies? Do you see how It will never change Its tune? And how that will ultimately serve to your advantage?

You *can* do it. The Demon lies to you, you know this for certain; I've already proven it to you, and It's lying Big Time when It says you can't talk to anyone about this. It knows if you do, yet another chunk of Its power is going to disappear, a really big one, and the Panic buttons are getting pushed, and pushed hard. The Demon is still trying that tired old tirade, "I AM You. You can't tell them about Me, that would look bad *for You*. It will only show them the ridiculous, disgusting, idiotic fool you are!"

Do I need to remind you when It's lying now? Nahhhh, you're getting good at recognizing Its methods now too, aren't you?

So here's how you start, you say, "I want to talk about something that is really hard for me to discuss." Right away, you've admitted your intention to begin a discussion, and your feelings of difficulty that may arise due to it. Now you don't have to worry, your friend already knows you're about to dish something big, and that you chose him or her because you knew they could listen with the best ears.

For me, when the conversation itself began, it was my friend and coworker Kelly and it was during our lunch break. I told her I had been reading a book, about Eating Disorders (I could barely say the words), and that the book made me start thinking about things... about myself. I was frightened beyond belief, my hands were shaking as I clutched them in my lap; every instinct seemed to be screaming, "Stop! Stop now! Change the subject, *quick!*"

Instead of stopping, I told Kelly, "There is a Voice inside my Head, and It tells me bad things, all day long. It tells me I'm not good enough. It tells me I'm a horrible person, no matter if I've done a thousand good deeds that very day. It makes me hate myself."

Kelly nodded, and folded her hands, looked me directly in the eyes, and said, "Alissa, I have the Voice too. Please... go on."

We were late getting back to our desks that day. The tears we both shed were golden prisms of Infinite Light.

You are not Alone.

How many of your sisters that you know out in your own immediate sphere do you think are silently suffering from this Demon, the same as you and I? Pick any number and quadruple it. The statistics state 2.4 million Americans suffer from some form of this disease. That number doesn't even account for the hidden ones. The sad fact is, most often eating disorders can be hidden for many years, they don't always evidence themselves in outward appearance (especially bulimia) and they can infest us, undetected, with a lifetime of Pain.

"Hoops? What Hoops? I don't know what you mean, I don't have any 'Hoops.'"

The scale. Put it away. *Throw it away.* And don't go and buy another when you panic about it after the trash gets picked up. The calories? Don't look. Don't need to look, you already know? Then when the Demon tells you, "That's 500 calories, you fat bitch," you can tell It right back, "Yep, 500 for me, and none for you, you sick lying bastard!"

The Rules... you know your own Rules. Start to discard them. One by one. What if the off limits foods weren't off limits? What if butter on your bread, fat on starch, gave you comfort and nourished you, as nature intended? What if you no longer skipped desserts? Ever!

What else, what other Hoops? The False Fronts. It's time to let them fall away. When will you stop pretending? And once you stop pretending, there's nothing left to be, nothing left to do, but to be the Real You. Begin to discard them, now. Today. Don't put the mask on. Frown instead of smile, cry instead of grin.

What's wrong with being authentic? The Demon said you were forbidden from knowing another's compassion, therefore you weren't allowed to show Pain... that was Its demand so you would remain Its emotional thrall. The Demon is a lying sack of... yeah, that.

When is the A+ finally plussed enough? When you learn not to care about satisfying the Demon. When you can accept yourself as having faults, and yet realize you are a good person who knows how to Love. When you see the Demon for all Its lies. When you can feel comfort eating graham crackers with your afternoon tea, and eat them all without making a single bargain with the Demon.

Only you know when you're ready, and which Hoops you can let go of, and when. Maybe it's only one, and maybe it's only for one day. But one day makes tomorrow easier, trust me. It really *really* does. (And no... if you keep listening to your Demon, you will *never* be ready, because It doesn't want this change to *ever* happen).

Suffering in silence feels hard, but really, it's easy. It's cowardice; unwilling to deal with the fear of rejection and humiliation, we do nothing, say nothing. Rule Number One. We pretend until the end. But, when you stop pretending that a magic number on a scale will make you feel better, what is left inside? What falls off, what dies if you don't need to be "skinny" in order to be okay?

And, more importantly, what remains?

It's not easy, it's not… but breaking the Silence is crucial. It is the most powerful way you can dissociate your Authentic Self from your Demon, your very best emotional and material weapon. You give power to the belief of being separate from this Demon when you say aloud, to someone else, "This is what I've been doing, and this is what I've been thinking… and this isn't the real me. It's this terrible thing that people call an 'eating disorder' and I really don't like it. I want to be rid of it. I need your support, even if all you do is listen to me ramble."

In AA, they have sponsors. A sponsor is there for you to reach out to when the going gets really tough, when you feel tempted to slip into your old habits. Find yourself a sponsor; it may be the same person you first decided to tell your problem to. It may be your best friend, your boyfriend, your sister. It may be a professional counselor. Whoever it is, tell them what you need them to be… maybe you just need someone to talk to, someone to listen without judging or trying to "fix" you. Maybe you need an outside objective source for feedback.

There was a time when I was growing stronger that I could admit to my husband that I "had a problem with weight issues." The words sounded so clinical and superficial. But they were the best I could do. I had put the scale in the garage—something he had noticed but chosen against commenting on. And I told him I may need his help if I begin to look too thin and I couldn't really trust myself to make that decision (I knew my Demon was still too loud inside my head, but I was working on it).

I asked him to replace the scale as my point of view. And it worked wonderfully. I honestly don't remember how long the scale stayed in the garage; it was at least six months or more. When we moved it back into the house, by that point I had grown strong enough to remove the Hoop of checking the scale every time I went to the bathroom (or showered, or ate, or any of it any more). In time, I forgot it was even there.

But while "recovering," I knew my perspective was too screwed up, and I knew I needed an outside source to help me see myself. "I may seem kinda crazy for a while," I apologized. Crazy? No… crazy is living your life with this Demon in your head that screams ugly-nasties all day long and deciding that such a thing can not only be tolerated, but obeyed without question.

Getting someone to listen? Looking for someone outside the battle who could help? That wasn't crazy. That was the sanest thing I could have done. But yes, you will feel the Fear. That's normal, I promise.

Break the Silence. Words have wings. They can help to set you free.

I cannot tell you when you will be ready to start eating again. I cannot be the one to take the Hoop of purging after every meal away from you. I cannot fix your mind enough to convince you that being "thin" has nothing to do with feeling loved, or accepting yourself. I cannot *make* you turn against your Demon, instead of accepting Its litany of demands and lies.

These are *your* Hoops. *You* decide. *You* decide when to realize the need to control your body as an attempt to control your mind isn't working, and it never has. And *you* decide when it's the right time to hold your meal inside you, and not vomit it away, no matter how scared and uncomfortable you feel.

These can be very hard choices, and they require a lot of objectivity… which can be hard to find when you've listened to an abusive interior voice for a long period of time. Much like a victim of verbal abuse, it takes a while to un-do all the months or years of "tapes" you've had in your head, telling you negative things. These thought patterns take a while to change, but they *can* change.

A friend on a Tarot forum once said, "There are several inner voices we have. It is important to cultivate the right one." This is so beautifully succinct and just resonates for me. Khatruman understood the power of the internal dialogue, as well as what can happen when we learn to attune ourselves to the other voices our mind can speak in, the voices of our angels, our Teachers. Our Gods.

It is what we can hear inside our minds when the screams and insults of the Demon are finally squelched.

I said all along, I cannot walk your path for you. I can only show you the answers I found along the way that helped me.

There was a physical therapist I once knew, Alice, who told me that the body of one of her patients had just been found that morning. No sign of foul play, the police pulled the dead woman's body from her own car. The woman, Alice said, was an advocate against eating disorders, had professed to her own recovery, and had devoted her life to being a nutritionist and counseling women. She had given a lecture on nutrition earlier that very day.

She killed herself. Suicide. The Demon won. She kept up her every False Front, and by God, she fooled them all didn't she, with her lectures about proper diet, and assurances of personal good health? It hurt when Alice told me of her. I felt guilty. I too had heard the news that morning of a woman's body that had been found, but Alice's tale made this headline a real person.

Someone like Me. Someone with a Demon. Someone who could have been saved, if she only knew how to save herself.

And she was just one, one of thousands, millions, which exist out there. They have No Voice. I know they can't Talk, their voices have been stolen, like Ariel and the evil queen in "The Little Mermaid." They want to speak but have no ability until the moment the spell is broken. And by Goddess, I wrote this book to try to be the Voice. To Speak Up and to tell you that you *do* have the power to break the evil queen's spell, all on your own.

I wanted to tell others what I've discovered about Demons before someone else became the next headline. I see you scoffing, "Not me, Alissa." Maybe you would never actually manage to check yourself out... but maybe you would.

Maybe you wouldn't even *want* to die, but the Demon found your Pain so delicious, It ate you up anyhow. You withered away, shrunken into nothingness, just the way It likes you, until you were gone.

Did you know... did you know that Terry Schiavo suffered from bulimia? Did you know that before the nation argued about her right to live or die in 2005, her coma began when her body went into shock from the electrolyte deficiencies that years of her bulimic abuse had caused? I don't think Terry meant to die either. But, her Demon meant to kill her with Its brand of kindness, and so It did. And then the Demon starved her to death, just as she wished for It too when she created It. She never gave herself another chance to change her mind. Her body was too far gone.

My dual Hatred of the Demon, and my need to continue defying It by breaking the self-imposed silence of Rule Number One is what prompted me to write this book. I cannot stand by and listen to yet another story of the Demon winning, not when I know I can *try* to help. To share the answers that I found, to try and show another the way out from the hell that they've been in.

Maybe it only helps one other person in the world... but then, maybe that person is you.

For the decade that I lived in this hell with my Demon, no one knew of my problems. For over 10 years I was able to hide much of what I did from everyone—from my parents, my coworkers, my husband, my friends, my fellow dancers, my sister. The Shame is so oppressive to live with, isn't it?

I haven't banished It for good. It's still there in me. I can't forget that. But It isn't driving my life, my thoughts, or my actions anymore. I've starved It to the point where It grew tiny and weak, and I am in control again. That's reaching the other side. That's the end of the road that we've been walking, together.

I took the cage the Demon used to lock up my Authentic Self, and in freeing her, I threw the Demon in instead, and locked It inside for good.

The only reason I come back to this horrible place is to try and help people, especially if someone is calling to me from inside the terrible Darkness of an eating disorder. And yet, just like I said, I'm only the tour guide out. I'll never leave your side. But, I can't make you walk forward. It's up to you. This is your fight, not mine.

Let go of your Hoops. You know they don't work anyhow. You know hurting yourself to be "thin" will never give you control over the Demon because those behaviors *came* from the Demon. You can only starve that nasty beast by learning to Love, and Love, and Love some more. You can even begin to Love yourself enough to let go of the Blame and the Guilt. And you can show yourself Love in the real world by removing the Hoops.

By eating again. By living again. By creating the perfect world for the little girl inside to take over. A world where she can play and be free. Every time you put down a Hoop, her hope grows.

The other day, my young son closed his eyes tight while playing a game with me. "Open my eyes!" he said, grinning.

"Only you can open your eyes," I giggled.

Only You can Open Your Eyes.

❧The Process of Recovery☙

"I'm just not hungry right now. I'm fine; I don't feel very well. I get sick when I travel. I'm angry, I'm upset; I don't feel like eating right now."

There is this awkward aspect to getting healthy again. Maybe you're reading this chapter, and you know you're still in the same mental space that you were when you read page one... you know in your heart that you aren't better (yet!) Or, maybe you are recovering, barely able to admit to yourself and others that yes, maybe I can become healthy again. You're not fully there, but you know you're on your way. An inch at a time.

Regardless of where you're at right now on this journey, let me show you the fast-forwarded version of eating disorder recovery. This isn't the pretty part. There are some social obstacles, you see. An alcoholic can avoid alcohol, that is, his vice... but we can't avoid food. Eating, no matter if we feel good, bad or indifferent to the task, is a necessary part of being a human. You are not going to be able to throw away your needle, like a junkie, and walk away from your old life.

But no one talks about what to expect *after* we've managed to wrestle the Demon into the cage in any of the self-help books out there. They don't tell us that *you* may know you're better, but the people around you may still treat you like you're not.

The day will come, if it hasn't already, when you will be saying to yourself, "Hellfire, I *did* it! I managed to beat the Demon! That's so freakin' awesome, I'm so proud of myself, I feel happy again!" And in your heart of hearts, you will *know*, "Yes! The Demon isn't deciding things any more." The Demon isn't calling you names. You aren't bartering with the Demon about calories or situps. The scale doesn't even enter your mind when you walk in the bathroom any more. You're Hoop-free! You really *really* are!

But... you see, here's where the tricky part shows up. Let's look at me; it's been nearly a decade since I last made myself throw up and/or starved myself as a means to punish my body, and thereby control my world. It's been a long time; I've had a while now to cage this Demon inside me.

But the funny thing with an eating disorder… some of the folks who love you, they get so scared. Early on, they may find it hard to believe you're actually better, *especially* if they were one of the ones who never even knew you were sick until you told them.

And the worst part is, although my Demon doesn't run things, the truth is It *is* back there, lurking and waiting for the day that I might fall into my old habits again. Into bad mental habits especially, It loves to work over my head when I'm feeling low; It knows my body is strictly off-limits, but sometimes It still tries to run things inside my head. I have to catch It when that happens, which I do, by using the same methods we've already discussed and have become second nature to me now.

BUT! The minute I would see the worried frown of someone I love when I pushed my plate away half-full, I feared what they were surmising. They assumed I'm behaving like I still have my eating disorder. Right then, they couldn't see inside my head any more than they could before when the Demon *did* call the shots. And I can't *make* them realize I really am better, but I just don't feel good right now.

Emotions affect the physical body. As humans, it is common for us to find eating less appealing when we are sad, angry, or depressed. You will know those days again in the future; despite being healthy you will become upset again. It's gonna happen. Be extra careful during those times. I tune in to my Teachers a lot when these hardships occur.

You are going to have to become your own advocate someday. Once you're on the other side, and you know how to love yourself again… you're not done. Later, much later, you're gonna need to be so strong in your mind and your heart that you can defend yourself when the recriminating looks that you no longer deserve continue to fall upon you.

There are long term consequences to entertaining the Demon by hurting yourself, you see. Bet your Demon never bothered to bring that up while It was busy creating the Pain of today, but there are consequences to an eating disorder—social ones, and physical ones—that won't show up for years. They show up when you're better, and in doing so, they will challenge you all over again. This too is the path.

In Tarot's Major Arcana, the Judgement card appears when the Fool's journey is nearly complete. It signifies the time has come to be reborn, to stand up and be who you really are; it shows how the necessary changes in your life are all behind you now—the Death card is all about irrevocable changes, such as Caging the Demon, but by this point... the change itself happened a long time ago. The binging was in your past; all the Rules are gone.

The Judgement card declares now is the time to simply *own* yourself, and your life. It is not about being judged, it is about realizing you are whole. Only your perception was compromised, due to the Demon's influence. The Real You is ready to stand up, and to joyously take control once more. This is her rebirth.

The card illustration by Pamela Colman Smith shows an angel blowing a trumpet, greeted by the souls around her. Without clothing, with nothing to hide, the souls' arms are lifted in joy and their expressions encompass ecstasy and wonder. In the Angel's presence, there is the ultimate form of recognition... by shedding the layers of falsehoods, we are spiritually naked and realize there is nothing to feel shame for.

No shame, no embarrassment, nothing left to hide. What does that really mean... to us? It means no more need for False Fronts, no need to keep pretending. It means no longer feeling guilty or shameful for eating food and keeping it inside you. It means shutting down the voice of the Demon until It is the one who is silenced and the Real You is the one who does the talking in her life once again.

The angel's trumpeting alarm calls to us within, and with her call, we seek to rise up... to exist in a state of benevolence and Love. Of authenticity and integrity. To live an existence that mirrors the Source, that sacred place from which our soul was made and seeks to spiritually evolve towards.

This is your path. This is what you lost sight of, but are finding within you once again. Just as you were meant to all along. You created this eating disorder from the pain you endured. Now, it's up to you to realize although you are Its creator, you do not need to be Its host. And you can be Its serial killer now too.

For too long, the two have masqueraded as one… the Demon and the Real You have lived a dualistic life, twisted into each other until you became one identity… one set of behaviors. A set united in its opposition against each other.

The word "integrity" is defined as the quality of being whole, undivided, and complete; by learning to reunite the divided halves of the eating-disordered psyche, the Demon versus the Authentic Self, you have learned to recognize and understand *your* authentic emotions as something distinctly separate from the Demon's impulses. In doing so, you have learned to dissociate yourself from your disorder and all the behaviors (the Hoops) associated with it in order be healed. *Healed…* not for a while, but for good.

Stop a moment and breathe deeply. With your eyes closed, picture yourself encased in bright, shining, glimmering, sparkling Light. Like a bubble, it surrounds you. Allow your emotions to shift as you bask in the presence of this Light a while before you open your eyes again.

Again, the Judgement card is *not* a card about judging yourself, or about being judged. The judging, the criticizing… those are the tools of the Demon. The Judgement angel is here to remind you that the Demon's reign is over. Noted Tarot scholar of the last century, Arthur Waite said, "It is the card which registers the accomplishment of the great work of *transformation* [my emphasis] in answer to the summons of the Supernal—which summons is heard and answered from within."[2]

The day will come when, for whatever reason, you're gonna get up from the dinner table to go to the restaurant's bathroom and a "look" will pass from one person to another as you leave the table. Silence, the Demon's Rule Number One. Your loved ones are playing the Demon's games, and they don't even know it.

And you may wonder, "Do I say something, do I not? Do I deal with their unspoken words of accusation when I know I'm finally blame-free and all I have to do is pee? Or do I pretend I didn't see it?" I just deal with it, and I don't open conversations that don't need to begin.

---

[2] Waite, Arthur E. The Pictorial Key to the Tarot (London: Rider and Sons, 1910) p. 148.

That is my choice. Only *I* know if I am sick; only I know if my Demon is in control or I am. So who cares what the rest of the world thinks?

This laissez-faire attitude is how I've learned to deal with the Demon's temptations. I've finally gotten well enough to feed myself regularly, forget about the scale completely, abandon all the old Rules, and to stop the name-calling; I can actually take care of myself very well. And I can defend myself... especially during the times when others might think I'm doing something wrong, and I know I'm not. I often defend myself by saying nothing that doesn't need said. Internally, I realize that no matter what the rest of the world may think, I know that I am Whole. I affirm this to myself as often as I need to. In this, I continue to keep the Demon's gag on tight.

The Demon would love to step in during any of those given moments and say, "They don't believe in you, and neither do I! Go throw up, go prove them right! That will fix them and their righteous attitude. You think you're over Me? Look how huge you are!"

Just looking for any opportunity to start up the Hate Train again, that Demon. Not gonna do it, Demon. Remember how comedian Dana Carvey would say that line as President Bush 41 on *Saturday Night Live?* "Naht gahnna dew eht...." That's me, talking to my Demon.

Only *you* know.... If the Demon's talking to you, only you know if you're gonna chose to listen. Others may make their guesses, but *you* have to be the one to take care of you.

I have a thin frame, I always have. Even when my Demon was in control, my weight never slid so dangerously low that folks could "tell." I had always been thin, and so a little thinner wasn't so noticeable. But it also isn't as noticeable now that I'm better either. My doctor confirmed I have an active thyroid, and I'm still thin. I weigh only slightly more than I did over a decade ago when my Demon ran the ship–except around the holidays, then I'm happy to say I gain the typical 10 pounds every year!

You can't look at me and know I'm "better" any more than you can look at a stranger on the street and know if they're suffering too. It can be hidden, especially bulimia (which comes in people of all sizes, not just bone-thin). That ability to hide the problem works for you when you are still the Demon's victim; it works against you as a survivor.

Learn to accept the metabolism and body frame you were born into in this life. Each day, when the Demon presents Its tantalizing images of bones and skin, see the child inside. Would you make her starve to become this? Or would you teach her to love the miracle of her body which is meant to program itself... not something to be controlled and despised.

The Demon's cage must be strong and Its gag must be kept tight. I'll give you another version of how the Demon would like to begin our deadly conversation again, it occurs from time to time in my life.

I like Diet Coke. I really do, and I always have. It's not the calories, I *like* the taste of Diet Coke—the new Coke with Splenda that tastes just like regular Coke proved that to me. I hate that stuff! But, I do *love* Diet Coke.

My Demon doesn't talk to me any more when I grab a Diet Coke with my lunch and yet, strangers feel that it's okay to tell me, "Oh yeah, like *you* need to drink something diet!"

For a moment, especially early on in recovery, you flinch inside. You freeze. You wait for the internal voice of the Demon to tell you what to say, how to react. But the Demon...? Freaking bastard, I gagged Its ugly mouth, locked It in a cage and threw away the key.

So *I* have had to learn how to deal with these moments by myself. This judgment that I didn't ask for, this judgment I have worked so hard to rid myself of. Yet strangers feel justified in judging me....

How do I deal? You learn to let it slide right off your back. My Demon takes these random comments as a moment to try to gain control once more, "Don't believe her for a minute, you fat cow, you're exactly the kind who needs to be drinking a diet! Look how huge your thighs...."

Shut Up Demon, I tell It. Visualize the gag and place it over the ugly mutt's mouth to silence It if I must. I take Its control away, like a parent scolding an errant child with a grounding. You're grounded, Demon...

go to your cage, stay there and don't make a sound! I take away Its voice, the way It once stole mine from me.

And, in real life, I pop the top, smile, shrug and say, "But I like Diet!"

Who cares what they think, it's what *we* are thinking in our own heads that matters. So who cares? The Demon will try to make us care, but we can't give others that power over us. "Who Cares?" is the name of a ballet that George Balanchine choreographed after Suzanne Farrell, perhaps his greatest muse, was released from the New York City Ballet. Letting go is the hardest part. Letting go of caring about It. It's so much easier said than done. That's why I'm taking the time to tell you about it now.

The Demon may try other forms of shapeshifting on you as well; outside incidents can trigger the Demon, rattling Its cage. A boss' harsh words, or a parent's unasked for criticism may give the Demon a hook—a way to try and get back in again. Be wary of It, and do not allow It to make the decisions in your life. Not in how you eat. Not in how you react after you eat. Not in how you think of yourself. And certainly not your ability to remember your Divinity, and to react with loving kindness and positive intentions, even to those who cause you distress.

Here's another aspect of being recovered, and yet being challenged by the choices of before. I have some bad habits. Bad is defined as being detrimental to the overall health and wellbeing of my body. You may have bad habits, even when you're recovered. Me, I forget to eat. Some folks will understand that, and others never do, but it's true. I *forget* to eat.

I can sit down with coffee, skip breakfast as usual, get busy on some writing until lunch, drink a protein shake, jump up and down to attend to my son 101 times, and then the next thing I know... it's almost time for my husband to come home and I've got a headache. DUH! Alissa, you forgot to eat again. The shake was hours ago, and wasn't enough for your body.

I don't do this every day, but I do have these kinds of bad habits. I have to watch myself, I try to catch myself.

My friend Joanne talked to me often of her "Inner Physician," one of her Teachers who would step forward during times when she was weak and needed help taking care of her physical body. I liked the idea and called on my own Inner Physician to come forward during my prayers, and mine showed up. All of us can do this, I firmly believe that. Each of us has these guides, these Teachers, but as I said before, it is up to *us* to begin that dialogue.

The inner dialogue between a Guide can be open and ongoing when you invite it to be so. Remember that analogy I mentioned earlier? Spiritual guides are like a reference collection, the book only works if you open it up. Otherwise it sits mute on the shelf until the day you discover it.

"What does a Guide sound like then; it just sounds like your own thoughts, right? So how do you know it isn't just the Demon's voice you're still hearing?"

For me, and others I've talked to, the voice of a Guide does come through as part of the interior monologue... yet this voice, unlike the one that says, "You forgot to get the dry-cleaning," speaks in a way that carries more authority. It is a reliable and soothing voice, and brings only loving messages which calm me down and embolden my heart with Love.

You already know what it's like to live with a voice in your head. The Demon's. The Demon's voice is easy to recognize as distinctly separate from a Guide's because the Demon's messages spread Pain. An Inner Teacher does not spread Pain; an Inner Teacher operates from the Source, and the Source is Love. By examining the nature of the messages you receive, you can easily tell the difference between the Demon and the calm voice of Spirit if you hear messages from within.

As Waite said, it is the Supernal call which we hear and answer from within that must be undergone. It is not a path of Pain any more, but one of self-recognition, kindness and Love. By turning down the Demon's volume, by arguing It into the box and locking It there for good, you can turn up the volume for the other voices who can help you instead. The Voices of your Angels.

If you choose to open yourself to the guiding presence within you, the voice of Healing and Wisdom, you will find you are not spiritually alone on this path back to recovery. You have help, both in the outside world with your family and friends, and in your inner world with your God, and your Guides.

My own Inner Physician (I don't use names for my Guides so much as labels which assist in categorizing how they interact with me) helps me watch for my bad eating habits. I have been known to drink protein shakes after my morning coffee to stop my blood sugar from crashing until lunchtime. Come lunch, I make a point to stop and eat. I carry a protein bar in my purse for the times when I'm running errands and I suddenly realize, "Holy moley, I forgot to eat earlier and I'm already so late, I don't have time to hit a drive-thru."

It does get easier, believe it or not. You are not Alone.

There will be times when you will face the agonizing sympathy of others, and you will have to love them enough to *forgive* them for the mistakes they make—for the things they might think or say. You can do that too. That day will come; it may be closer than you already think. And I'm telling you now, so when it does, you'll be prepared.

Once while telling a medical professional of my eating disorder so she could record it for my medical files, she said in response, quite genuinely, "Oh you poor thing."

"No!" I barked back, stronger than I probably should have. "Not 'poor thing,' it was the thing that made me the person I am today. Fighting it made me realize how strong I really am." Pity belongs to the Demon; to accept her pity would have been to open the Demon's cage, just a little bit. Another may pity your own struggle as well... be prepared to instruct the non-Demoned that their compassion is appreciated, but the Demon doesn't deserve even an ounce of their pity.

There are other prices I have had to pay for the choices my Demon made long ago, other consequences I never imagined I was creating while I starved for so long—I have been diagnosed with osteopenia, an early form of osteoporosis. Being in my thirties, there are no medications approved for someone as young as I to reverse the condition; if I was in my menopause, I'd have a half dozen to chose from. Today, I have myself, God, exercise and lots of calcium to proactively rebuild my body and restore to it what I once denied. But the human body absorbs the most calcium into the skeletal system during the late teens and early 20s. Right when I was often abusing myself the worst.

Osteoporosis happens when the body must learn to consume itself in order to stay alive... for years, my body ate at my bones in order to keep doing what I asked of it ("keep dancing, keep working, keep writing, keep performing, you lazy bitch, faster!") all while refusing to give myself food. The Demon would tell me how strong I was to deny myself, and I felt pride in my ability to withstand such deep hurt and yet hide my pain. While praising me for fasting, the Demon forgot to mention that even long after I managed to kick Its ass, my body would still be paying the price for those repeated acts. And there is no pride in having brittle bones.

I tell my body often how sorry I am for what I did in my ignorance while blinded by the lies of the Demon. I love my body, and it is a joy to say those words when once they seemed such an impossibility. I love every inch, every roll, every wrinkle, and every pimple... I no longer call my body names and treat it as something to be hated and despised. As something to be controlled. My body is beautiful, just as yours is. Only the Demon told us how ugly and imperfect and *fat* we were.

Here's another challenge that awaits many long after the Demon's reign is over, retreating bone mass in the skull can result in teeth which no longer have something to hold on to. Without a bit of tooth decay, your teeth can fall out when the bone mass of the upper and lower mandibles, your jawbones, have retreated due to massive overall bone loss in the body.

This image haunts me. It is the face of the Demon itself. A face so hungry, it has consumed itself until nothing left remains. Gaunt and toothless, it is unable to eat, or to fight. It is the face I refuse to see in myself, and fight with passion to help others avoid.

But I have to do more now to make up for the terrible amount of Bad that I did to my body long ago. I have to be proactive and extra-vigilant, mindful of my exercise and calcium intake.

I must use my *experiences,* as well as the *wisdom* I've gained; I must become the World Dancer.

In Tarot, the World card comes after Judgement. It's the final stop in the Major Arcana; it shows a time when we have reached the ultimate point of fruition. Like all endings, it is a beginning. The card shows a naked woman dancing in a veil, she exists in a state of rapturous understanding—she is like Lord Siva, dancing in her own ring but not one made of fire, one made of greenery and life. She is ready to become the Fool again, to begin her journey once more, but this time, she has the wisdom of her experiences behind her to see her through. She is not the naïve Fool who began this journey so long ago. And yet, because she is staring anew, she is.

And she is not alone; four guides are seen in the corners of the card. She is being powerfully assisted by the benevolent forces of the Universe in her endeavors. Her body is the message of hidden magic; her posture evokes not only Siva's cosmic dance, but the Kabbalistic Tree of Life. The bend of her arms and her knees play connect the dots to the positions of the 10 sephiroth… "every little thing she do is magic."

This is the point you will reach if you keep moving forward, if you do not give up hope, *ever!* Despite the bad days, despite the times you may backslide. This is the promise that the Universe has made to you, as one of the most special, uniquely gifted and beautiful souls to grace our planet… that you are a part of All. That Wholeness exists in macrocosm in the quantum physics of the Universe, and it exists in microcosm as *you.* The moment when you realize this, your soul is dancing, and it is effortless again. You remember what it is to rejoice. By uniting your mind and body, you can move with integrity—that is, with wholeness—towards the Source again, as we are all trying to do together.

Love doesn't hurt to give or receive any more. Not even to yourself. The Demon lied to you and told you you'd never feel Love again. But you don't have to listen or obey anymore. You know what It is, and you know how It works and why. You also know how to fight back, and how to usurp the Demon's power, how to knock It from the huge throne It has occupied in your mind and body for so long.

The only thing left is to stay the course and to give it time. Time. All lessons are learned in time. It took time for this thing to grow; it will take time for It to shrink.

Where you are, right now, is where you needed to be to learn the lessons only *you* could have taught yourself, taught to your soul. You have been blindfolded and gagged by the Demon, and told that you were lost. I have removed the blindfold and given you this book as a Flashlight of Truth to find your way back.

And, in time, as you move further and further away from the Demon's influence… you realize you *are* growing stronger. You were never truly lost, but you had to journey that deeply away from the Source, from Love, in order to obey the Demon's commands, which you mistook as your own.

Now, you've turned on your Flashlight, and you've turned around to go back. Back to normal. Back to healthy. Back to feeling Love again.

The fight grows easier, but it takes great willpower. When you're low, remember… you are not Alone. You can replenish yourself and your energy in the Source, however you understand it. That can be time spent in a temple or church, it can be time spent in prayer; it can be a walk in nature, and it can be time of yoga, mindful breathing and private meditation. Don't forget to replenish yourself in the Source of ultimate energy and Light. Your Demon has convinced you to hate the Light, scurvy cockroach that It is.

You are already a creature of the Light, one who is inherently beautiful and perfect. Answer the Judgement angel's trumpeting call and stand up to be who you really are. Move yourself closer to that World card, you know you're getting close now. The Flashlight's directions don't look so foreign any more, do they?

Only loving kindness contains the Demon. Acts of loving kindness keep your cage for It strong. Loving kindness to others is fine… but it's loving kindness to yourself that you need to work on the most. Watch for times when the bars seem to bend, when you're feeling under attack. Do not allow It to determine your reactions in those times, or any other.

You are in control, and You are not It. You are inherently a creature of Divinity. It is only by losing our awareness of our own Divinity that allows the Demon the atmosphere It needs to attempt to take control again.

But you are stronger, because *God* is stronger and you are God. Behave in compassionate ways that express your own grace and spirituality, to yourself and to others.

React with Compassion to all Things, *most especially to the Self,* and the World Reacts the same.

❧Love's Eternal Embrace❧

"Oh God Alissa I'm at the end of the book, and I totally understand everything you've just said, but shit! I've not changed! I still throw up every day. What do I do now?"

These are the hardest times... when we understand intellectually but our emotions have yet to shift. First, be patient with yourself, just as I've said in the last few chapters. You've already come a tremendously long way, stop and realize how much you've learned.

You once thought that the Demon was You, and You were the one who was hating herself and hurting herself, and You had no idea why. You once thought that obedience to the Demon and Its Rules would bring relief, which it never did, but as a good and obedient girl would, you continued to hurt yourself to try and achieve freedom through a false sense of "control." You once thought you could never feel Love again; the best you'd ever know in life was numbness and eternal Pain.

Take a moment to metaphorically turn around and see how far you've come in understanding the true nature of this "eating disorder," and in such a short time. Stop and reflect on your arsenal of weapons... your lessons here have taught you firstly that you and It are *not* one and the same entity, which the Demon never admitted as true, nor wanted you to realize.

Then you learned how to recognize the Demon's Voice, how to talk back to the Demon, and later how to fight back by removing Its Rules, Its Hoops. You know how the Demon came to be, It was born of your own Pain. And you know *why* the Demon created nothing but Pain for you to live with... so It could maintain the energy It needed to grow. You know how to deny this Demon the Pain and Hate It needs to keep thriving inside your head; in doing so, you can starve It and deprive It of Its power in your life, not for a while, but for good.

The mental and physical self have suffered enough, and those battlefields have their share of wounds, but those wounds *do* heal. In time. If you are still bleeding inside, stay strong. Keep fighting until It is in Its cage, and *believe* that day will come, no matter what. Believe with all your heart that you are dragging your poor, tattered self back to the

Light, inch by terrible inch, with the Demon clinging to your heels and trying every moment to get you to stop.

It took me a long time before I really felt like I was "better." It took bad days along the way, and months of good days wiped out with one bad one... it takes more time for your body, mind and soul to complete this journey than it does for you to read this book.

Set your intentions every day; every meal, every bite, react with loving kindness. Not just for others, but for yourself too. Remember the little girl inside that you are protecting during the times when you still cannot give unconditional love back to yourself. Give it to her. In time, once the Demon is put away, she will merge with you... and you will be Whole once more, just as you were when your journey began in this life.

While I was traveling years ago, I noticed a *Newsweek* cover article with the compelling image of a young girl and the words, "Fighting Anorexia" emblazoned across her beautiful, young and unsmiling face. The irony of seeing this during the week of Thanksgiving, the holiday when we celebrate the bounty of life, did not escape me. We who suffer from an eating disorder live as a miser would during the holidays, operating under the logic of deprivation and self-punishment, much as Scrooge did before Marley and his ghosts arrived.

The article broke my heart. I could only read it in snippets it was so hurtful.

You see, the problem doesn't go away; it just grows quiet by society's standards. Today it's a headline, tomorrow it's back under the rug. But it doesn't go away. And it doesn't obey society's rules, so gee... all the tired theories like "stopping your body from menstruating" suddenly break down. Why? Because they were never true to begin with. The girls in this article were startlingly young, and some had yet to even begin their womanly cycles. Despite what the psychologists may think, these rules of theirs are *not* the Rules that apply; they are *not* the Demon's Rules.

The Demon had found a way, somehow, to already land these children, these precious baby girls, in Its ugly hooks. When I read one's description of hearing nasty voices in her head... there was that same sinking feeling. The feeling I get every time I hear of a sister who is suffering, and still does not know how to recognize the Voice of the Demon. A sister who is still operating under Its most insidious Lie... that she and It are One and the Same.

The article tells of frustrated parents met with bouts of vicious anger, followed by obstinate silence to their attempts to plead and negotiate. It hurts me to read... those parents don't understand, they aren't talking to their child. They're talking to their child's Demon, and what they see is only the tip of the iceberg. The rest of the Demon is lurking deep inside, growing maliciously as the Hate around It provides the nourishment for It to thrive.

And there again is the grand irony... the Demon's ever-changing false theories and identities help to keep It hidden in our society, corruptive and elusive. The *Newsweek* article tells us the disease is manifesting in a growing number of the very young; the ABC broadcast tells us the disease is afflicting more and more of the middle-aged and aging baby boomers. Theories about body image miss the point entirely. They only give power to the metaphor of the Demon's lies, while It slips outside the logic of others and laughs as It sinks Its talons inside all who fall victim.

I often don't want to talk about the fact that I've had an eating disorder. "I don't wanna go there," ya know? You get to a point where you've conquered It, and you're beyond It at last... and you don't want to ever bother even *thinking* about how ugly and dark and bleak your life was for so long. You just want to start over. Build on Love and Compassion, and forget the rest.

But I do go back there. I go back when I hear the cries of someone who is lost in that hell, and is reaching towards me. And the only reason they know to reach for me is because sometime prior I had volunteered, yet again, "that I used to have an eating disorder." They heard me say the words they couldn't yet speak, and then they dared to reach out and whisper, "How? How did you do it?"

I go back to try and throw them a rope, because I know they're going down, and this isn't the third time... this is the 30th time, and it's getting harder and harder to resurface. This one really *could* be it.

And so I have to keep saying it, "I had an eating disorder," because I know all too well that so many of the sufferers are obeying Rule Number One, You Cannot Say Anything. They need someone else to somehow open that forbidden conversation for them in order for their lives to heal. Someday, when you are better you may be ready to help another one of our sisters, to do the same for someone else in your own life. If not, that is your highly respected, personal choice. Each of us fights our Demon as we know we must.

Time has passed since I began this writing this book, and again, it's the holidays. Once more, I turn on the TV and hear reports on the problem of anorexia and young women. The holidays and its the celebratory feasts seem to spur regular interest in those who suffer from "eating disorders." Undetected, there behind the newscaster's monologue, if you listen you can hear the Demon's malicious cackle—It taunts me and tells me I can do nothing to stop It. It laughs and says how I may be free, but It will find more, many *many* more beautiful people, and It will twist them into the grotesque and hideous monster that It is.

While writing this book, there have been months of days where I simply have no wish, no desire, to go back to the tired subject of "how I got better." There is the Demon, shapeshifted and waiting, telling me that I will fail, that no one will ever read these words, that I have no right to dream, to aspire. That I have no right to believe I can help another person. That I can never truly beat It.

Love is stronger; Love is higher, and Love will carry these words I type today to the pages you read them upon tomorrow. Hope will deliver us where we need to be... me and you. Yes, there is the reason why I can't just forget about this book, I can't just let this go. Because I know all too well the Pain you're living in while smiling smiling smiling to the rest of the world... and I love you too much to pretend it doesn't matter.

I love you because I was once you, and we are All One.

So it does matter. I've never met you, but *you* matter to me. Your Pain matters to me, because I know you're here on this earth for better things than what your Demon has taught you to do. Surely there is more for you to accomplish in your lifetime than creating an over-reactive gag reflex, or the ability to wrap your arms around yourself and squeeze so tightly you can force the hunger pains to go back in. Brittle bones, vomiting blood, teeth decayed from stomach acid or dropping out of your skull from lack of bone mass, and a burning, thrashed esophagus weren't what you started this life with the intention of creating.

I can't give up. And neither can you. We have to believe, together. We have to do this, because it's what we were put here to do.

So, the choice is yours. I told you all along, I couldn't fight your fight for you. It's up to you. When do you tell It that you know being "thinner" does not equate to making Its accusations and lies stop, which is really all you ever wanted anyhow?

And if you don't need to be "thinner," you don't need to keep starving. Or purging. Or hating yourself for eating a normal meal. The behaviors drop away. The emotions connected to the behaviors are also discarded. And yes, it will take time.

You said, "I want control." You meant, I want to control this Demon and I don't know how. I've shown you how. You said, "I need to be perfect." You meant, I need to feel good about myself again. I've told you the Real You is a creature of Light that is already so beautiful and perfect and full of Love, the Demon can't even stand to have her around, so he threw her in an oubliette and hoped you'd forget about her.

You said, "I want to be thin." You meant, I want to like myself again. And you starved yourself to try to make that happen. The act of denying yourself made you feel "strong," any actions which caused Pain for the Demon to feed from were encouraged and nothing else was allowed to grow inside. Your painful emotions about your every scrap of food became the Demon's banquets; you didn't know why you kept hurting yourself so badly, but now you do.

You said, "I wish someone understood how much this hurts." And this book came to be in your hands, and Alissa showed up to hold you tight, to stroke your hair and to give you this Flashlight to help you find your own way back out.

Can you imagine what you'd be doing if you didn't have your Demon to entertain every minute of every day? Can you imagine how much more energy you'd have to give to other things, good things, if you didn't have to plan your day around meals and purging times? Can you imagine the person you'd see in the mirror if you removed the Demon's blinders at last, just as I've taught you to?

I know it won't happen until you're ready. I know it won't happen in a moment, even if you declare, like Spongebob, "I'm Ready!" I know it takes time. I know there are bad days.

But I know you *can*. You're stronger now than when we first sat down together. And look at your eyes, you no longer squint when we shine our Flashlights, our beacons of Truth, for others to see us by.

And me? I'll just keep talking, and I'll keep writing. And even during the days when I wanted to avoid the issue, I've kept at it in the hopes that someday, somehow… this message will reach You. The one who needed to hear this the most. This is my message in a bottle; I cast it and do not know who will read my words, but trust that Spirit will deliver the message for me, somehow….

The girl who uncorked the bottle is You. The girl who grabbed the rope and began pulling herself to safety, inch by terrible inch, with all her determination and might… it's You.

You don't need someone else to save you from yourself… you don't need a boyfriend, best friend, baby, husband, child or parent to rescue you from you.

You're *not* fighting yourself. You're fighting your Demon. And it is, most certainly, a battle only *you* can fight. But you're not helpless, and you're not ignorant about It anymore. I've given you my best arsenal of defense, and the Flashlight is on High. God is always with you, and you are always with God. If you can't believe in God, then believe in goodness… believe that you are already a Good Person. Without denying yourself anything, you are already a better person than your stupidass Demon would ever let you realize.

So you have to be the one to pull yourself back to safety. I'm throwing you the rope, and encouraging you to hang on–keep showing up on your end, keep at it the best you can, each and every day. It takes Faith. Faith in yourself, and if you possess a spiritually-minded heart as I do, Faith in the Divine. Faith in your *own* Divinity—and the realization that you are no different than God; you are *of God*, as well as part of a greater constellation of existence that each of us shares with one another in our world.

While writing this, the image I see inside is of Anne Frank before the end of her life, not locked in the attic but throwing notes over the walls of the concentration camp in which she was being held during her last days, in a blind desperate hope that someone would hear her... somehow. She never knew her diary would be found and the world would know her name. And she couldn't see over the walls that enclosed her; she couldn't be sure if her words of Hope from inside the prison camp would ever be delivered. If anyone would find them on the other side.

My words have been heard by you, and I am hearing, right now, your voice that was silenced by the Demon. I recognize your struggle, as well as your ability to defeat It. I am rejoicing in the knowledge that your Authentic Self will step forward once again to run the course of your life, that she is already tentatively doing so, and that every day you will teach her how to be strong while you create for her a world of beauty and Love. Your Demon taught you strength, and you can use that strength of character against It.

Take back your power, day by day, and while doing so, give It less of you in return. Less Anger towards yourself. Less Hatred of your reflection. Less Pain upon eating. And watch It die. If you're like me, you may get a certain delicious satisfaction at the notion of your Demon suffering, just as It convinced you to hurt and endure suffering yourself for so very long. I have no compassion for Demons.

Each of us can see the same little girl inside of us who was hurt so deeply when she was defenseless and innocent; she is the same wonderful little girl who has wanted to "make everything perfect" for everyone else, to try to make others happy in a vain attempt to fill the wound inside of her.

There is a way to feel full again without emptying yourself completely to do it.

You may feel completely incompetent on some days. You may feel an emotional wreck as the battlefield rages in your mind for the victor over your body. When you think back to the event that began this long downward spiral into hell, realize how old you were when it first occurred. In many ways, you are still that age… still that young girl who is learning her place in the world. You may be 18, but feel 13 in your perception and emotional reactions. You may feel 15, even if you're 26, in how you solve the problems that inevitably occur in your life as you recover, day by day.

This is normal. You will not take as long to "grow up" in real years. You are not the person you were then, and every day you are taking more steps away from that which you once were. Your emotional control will have to grow up with you, but it won't take as many years to catch up with your physical years, I promise.

Why? Because as you learn to face It, you gain back the power. And when you gain back the power, you realize You Are In Control, and not the fear. Not the anger and rage, not any more.

You are.

And with that glorious realization comes the epiphany that by being In Control of the Demon, you are no longer afraid to look at It. The more you have looked at It with me while using this Flashlight, the less fearful you became. And when there's less fear, there's less drive to continue acting out the coping mechanisms that the Demon taught you… the starving, the purging. It becomes easier to walk away from all of it… for good. The magic happens inside, and we answer that call we hear from within.

To just let It go.

Because You are Not It. You never were. Only It told you so, and It lies.

Lots of folks might have gone right back to the silence, unable to cope with the fear of facing the Demon, and suffered, maybe until death. Many of our sisters and brothers have died from their Demons.

But You grabbed this book and said… not Me.

You are not Alone.

The Demon… Isn't… ME!

You are Not Helpless against It.

The Real You is made of Love.

You *are* In Control.

Only You can Open Your Eyes.

React with Compassion to all Things, *most especially to the Self*, and the World Reacts the same.

You are Loved, and You are made of Love.

www.ingramcontent.com/pod-product-compliance
Lightning Source LLC
Chambersburg PA
CBHW030025290326
41934CB00005B/485